AF744009

Gastrointestinal Stomas

Edited by Vincenzo Neri

Published in London, United Kingdom

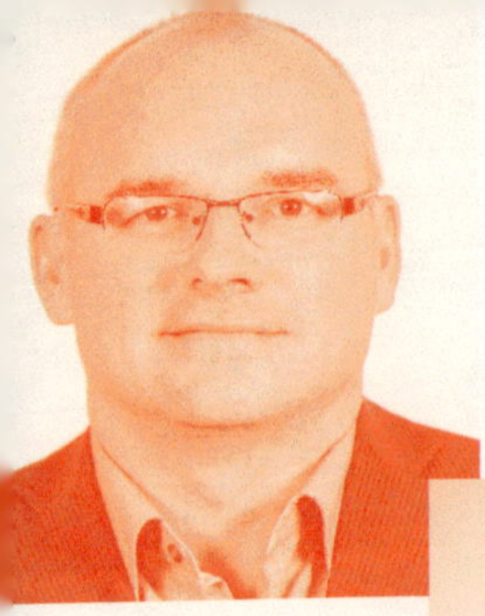
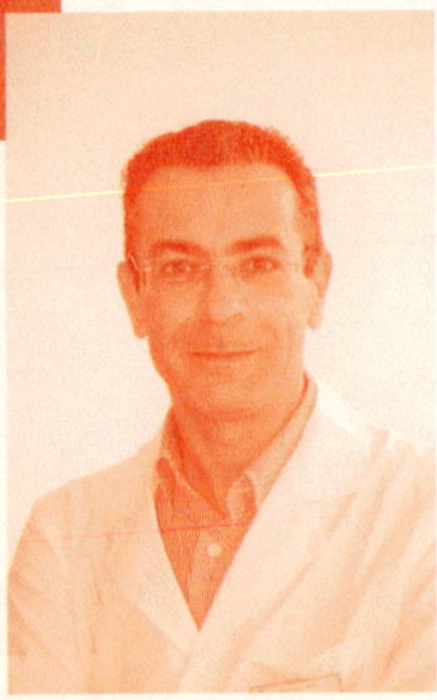
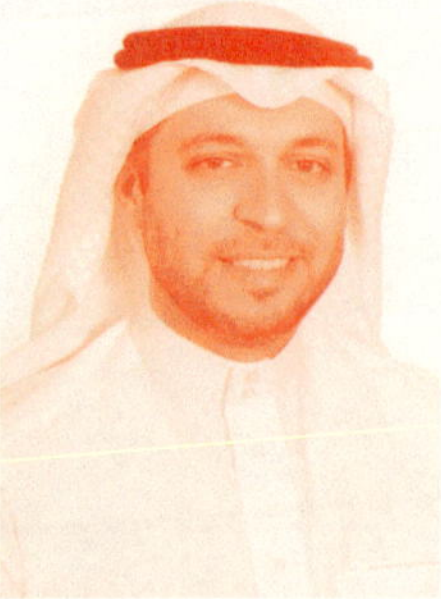
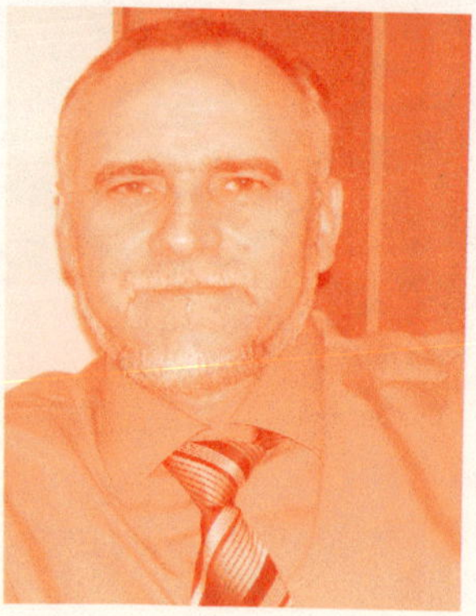
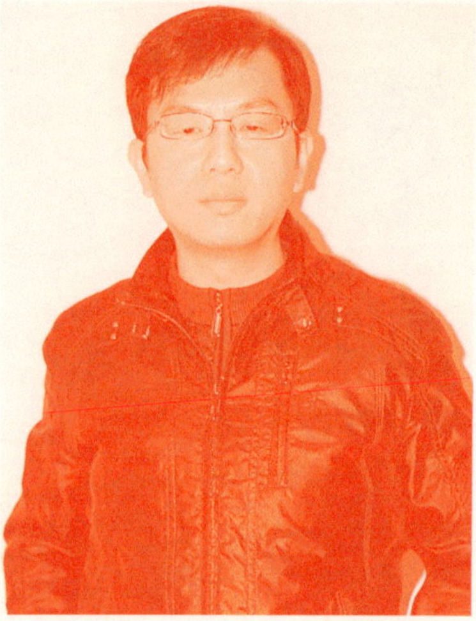
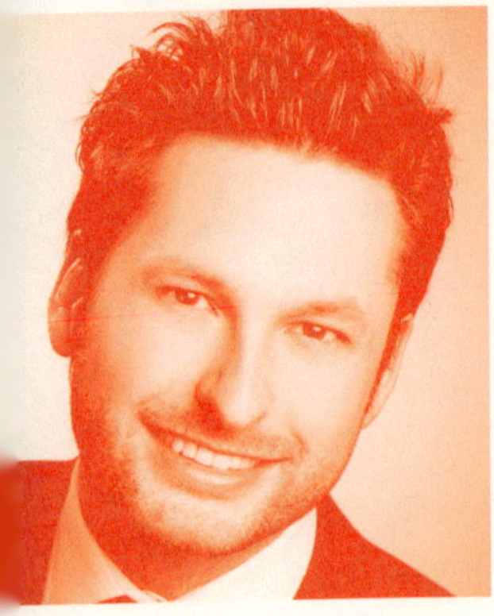
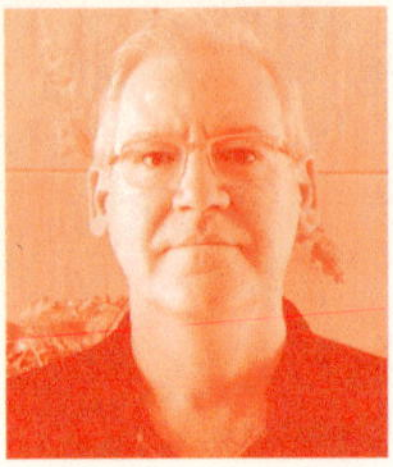

IntechOpen

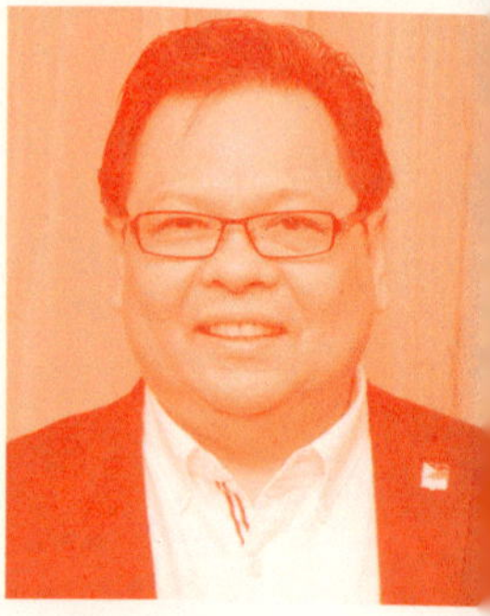
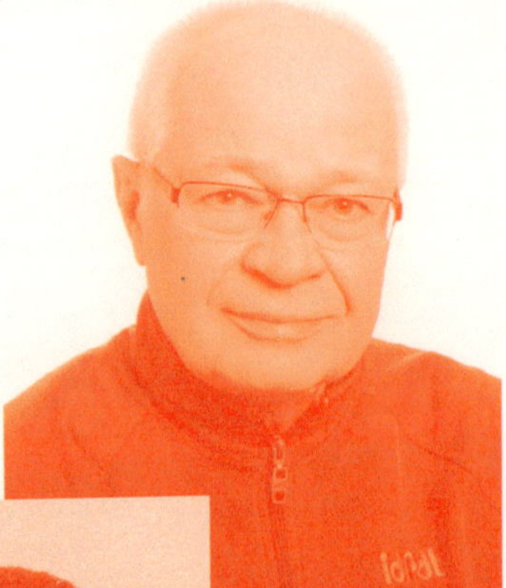
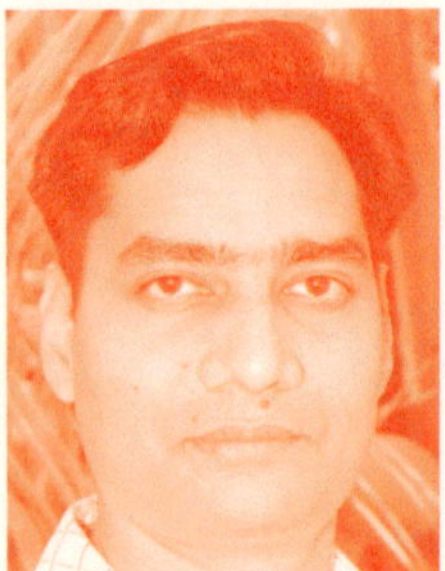
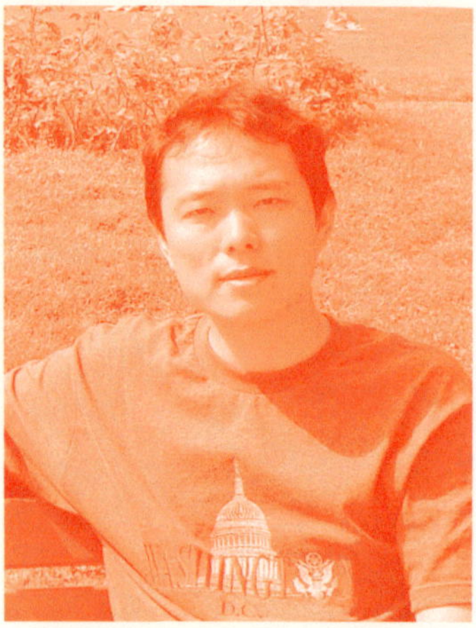
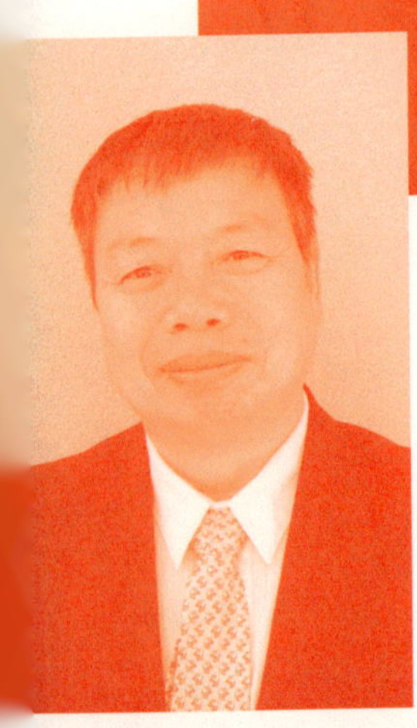
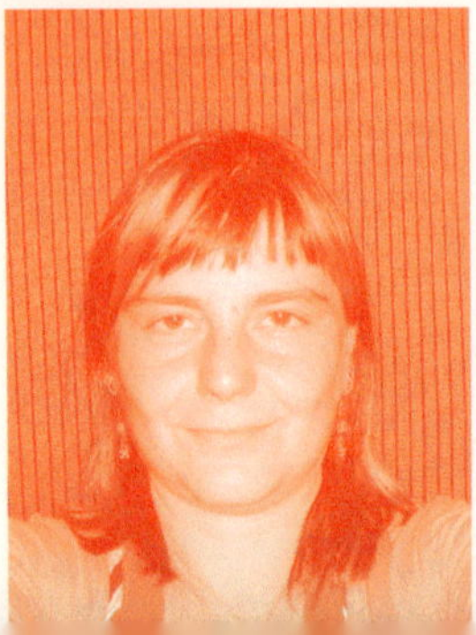

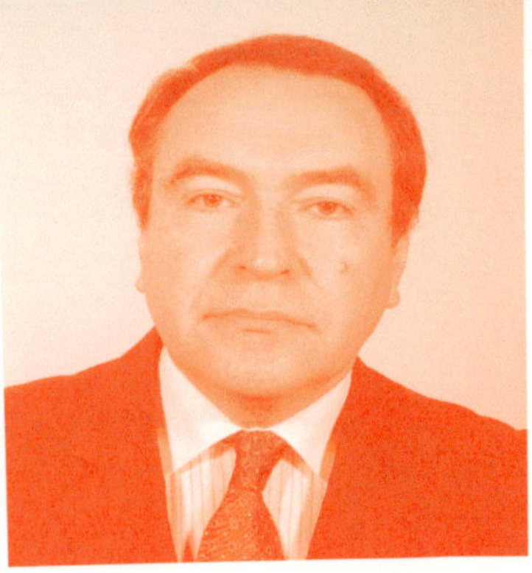
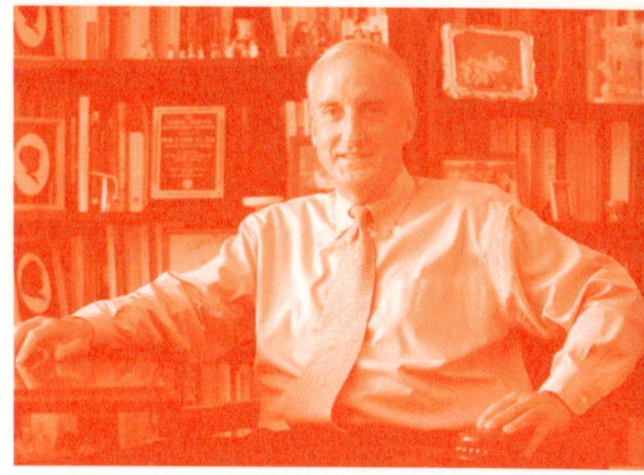
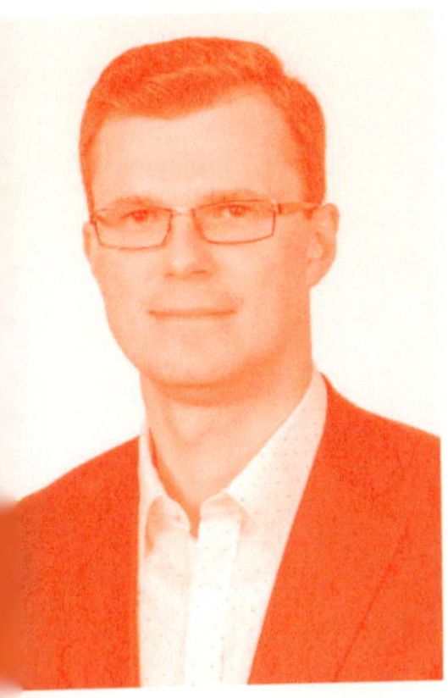
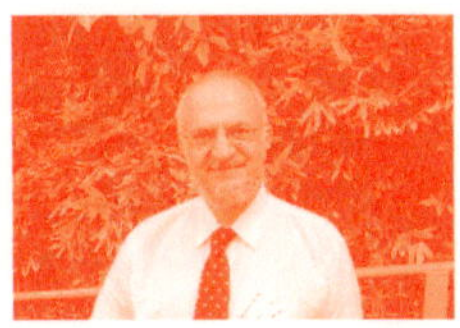
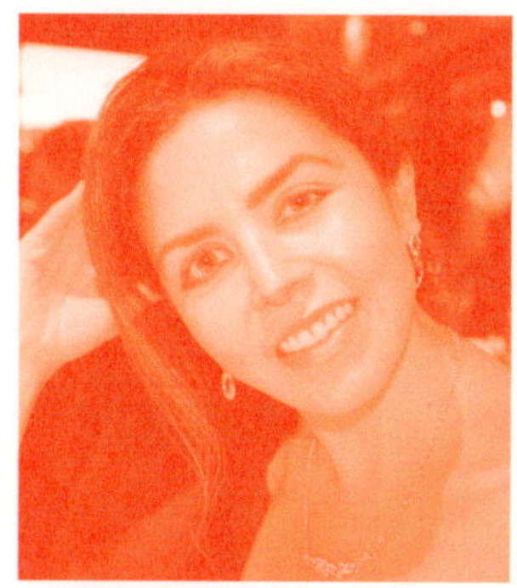

Supporting open minds since 2005

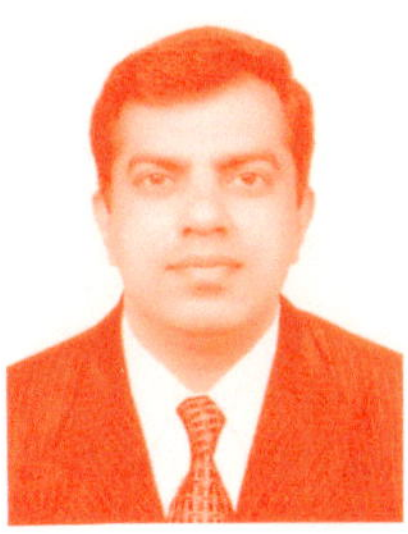
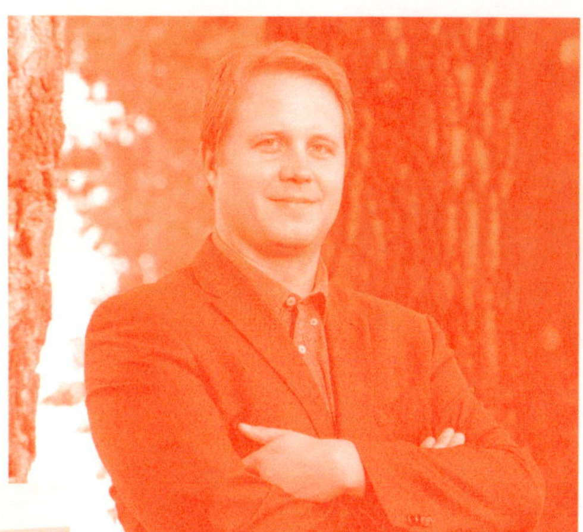
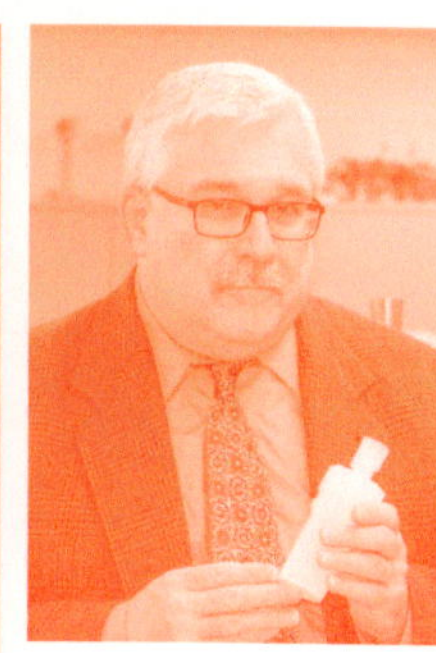
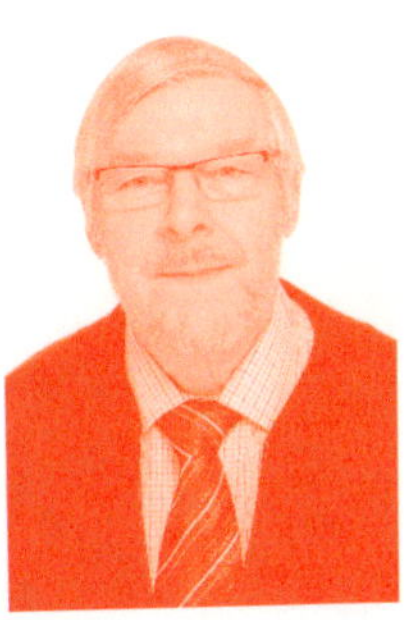
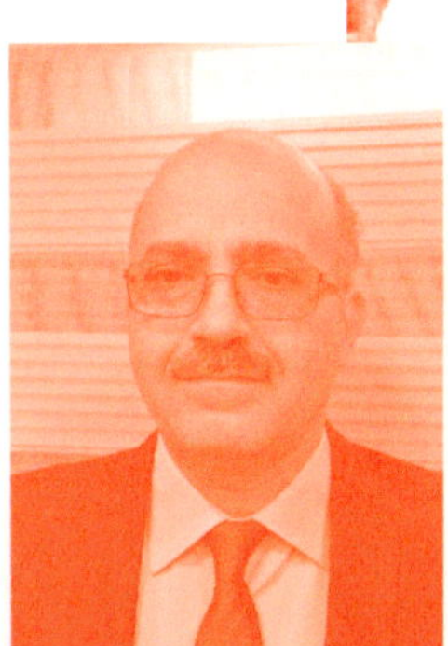
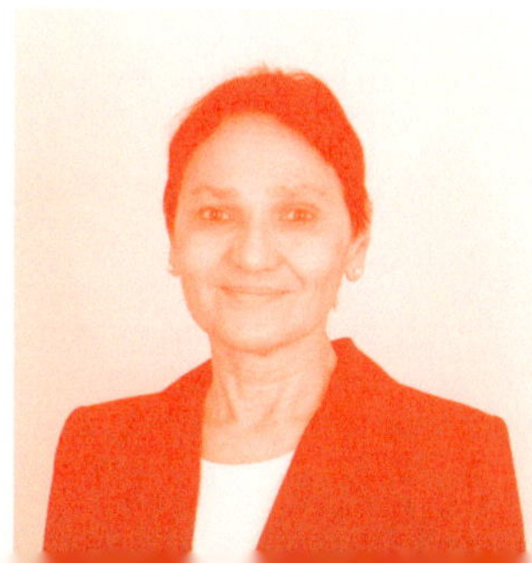
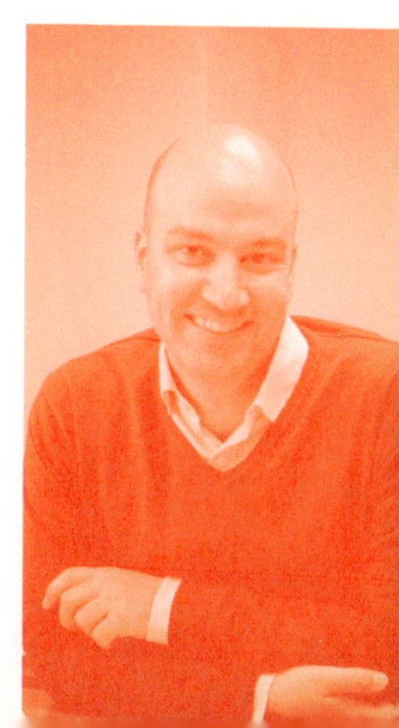

Gastrointestinal Stomas
http://dx.doi.org/10.5772/intechopen.78816
Edited by Vincenzo Neri

Contributors
Masaki Fujioka, Reihaneh Padidarnia, Mahsa Khodadoostan, Ahmad Shavakhi, Alireza Shavakhi, Mehdi Ahmadian, Hristo Ilianov Iliev, Mila Dimitrova Kovacheva-Slavova, Todor Asenov Angelov, Borislav Vladimirov, Hristo Yankov Valkov, Ali Bedran, José Renan Cunha-Melo, Marcela Monteiro Pinheiro, Jane Andrea Vieira Novaes, Francielle Profeta Rodrigues, Paula Martins, Ana Magdalena Bratu, Constantin Zaharia, Vincenzo Neri

First published in London, United Kingdom, 2019 by IntechOpen
IntechOpen is the global imprint of INTECHOPEN LIMITED, registered in England and Wales, registration number: 11086078, 7th floor, 10 Lower Thames Street, London, EC3R 6AF, United Kingdom
Printed in Croatia

British Library Cataloguing-in-Publication Data
A catalogue record for this book is available from the British Library

Additional hard and PDF copies can be obtained from orders@intechopen.com

Gastrointestinal Stomas
Edited by Vincenzo Neri
p. cm.
Print ISBN 978-1-78984-185-5
Online ISBN 978-1-78984-186-2
eBook (PDF) ISBN 978-1-83968-002-1

For EU product safety concerns:
IN TECH d.o.o., Prolaz Marije Krucifikse Kozulić 3, 51000 Rijeka, Croatia, info@intechopen.com or visit our website at intechopen.com.

Meet the editor

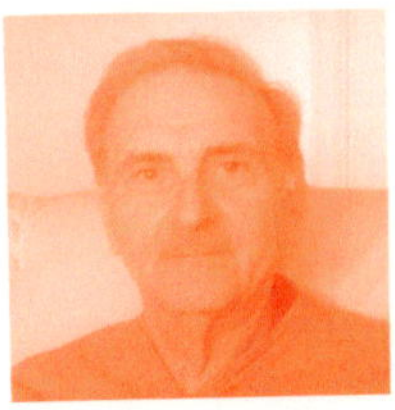

Vincenzo Neri was born in Bari, Italy, on March 15, 1946. He was Full Professor of General Surgery at the Department of Medical and Surgical Sciences at the University of Foggia (2002–2016). He was also Director of the Division of General Surgery (1997–2016) and Director of Residency at the School of General Surgery, Policlinic University of Foggia (2008–2016). He retired on November 1, 2016. He graduated in 1970 in Medicine and Surgery at the University of Bari, where he carried out a great part of his academic activity. Vincenzo Neri was Assistant Professor from 1974 to 1982 and Associate Professor from 1982 to 2001, both at the University of Bari. He obtained the diploma of "Maitrise Universitaire en Pedagogie des Sciences de la Santé" from the Université Paris-Nord Bobigny. In the ERASMUS-Program 2010–2011 at the University of Gent, Belgium, he developed a seminary on "Cystic tumours of the pancreas." He was the President of the Course of the Degree of Medicine and Surgery, University of Foggia, from 1996 to 2002, and was Director of the Department of Surgical Sciences, University of Foggia, from 2002 to 2008. His research's interest and the object of his publications is hepatobiliarypancreatic surgery. Vincenzo Neri has authored more than 330 scientific papers and edited both national and international journals on the topic of sovramesocolic region surgery. He is a member of the following scientific associations: SIC, IHPBA, AISP, EASL, NESA, and SLS.

Contents

Preface

Gastrointestinal stoma is a therapeutic measure that has been evident for a long time but which retains its validity even among the great and overwhelming advances in clinical practice. Some technical details of the performance of stomas and the frequency of use of the procedure have dramatically reduced but the indications have not changed. Currently, the vast majority of gastrointestinal stomas are temporary. Surgical indications of gastrointestinal stomas in different sites of the digestive tract are based on various pathological conditions. Frequency of the employment of intestinal stomas has varied greatly as time passes, and is linked to evolutions of therapeutic perspectives. Furthermore, the surgical techniques had ameliorative modifications with changes in therapeutic procedures. Most intestinal stomas are temporary, with a program to restore intestinal continuity: emergency ostomy in particular cases of intestinal obstruction, some anastomoses such as coloanal or ileoanal needing temporary diverting ileostomy, and temporary feeding ileostomy. Great care is required in performing and treating ostomy, because the procedure is a fundamental part of the therapeutic program and involves the surgeon, the patient, and the nurse stoma therapist. The therapeutic commitment of ostomy is not limited to local control but involves the evaluation and treatment of general conditions in ostomy feeding and the balance of fluid and electrolyte depletion in cecostomy and diverting ileostomy.

The first section, "Stoma Care," consists of four chapters. The "Introductory Chapter: Role of Colostomy in the Colorectal Pathologies" shows synthetically the current use of colostomy as a complement to colorectal surgery, with the changes that have occurred. The chapter "Stoma Revision on the Flaps in Cases of Abdominal Wall Defect with Digestive Tract Rupture" exposes the very complex topic of incisional hernia with abdominal wall defect, involving intestinal stoma. Resolution of this technical problem comprises various and discussed surgical procedures. The chapter "Intestinal Ostomy Complications and Care" develops completely and clearly the planning of ostomy and the outcomes of intestinal stomas evaluating functional and anatomopathological complications. The chapter "Gastric Microbiota: Between Health and Disease" is very interesting. The chapter introduces the important theme of the change in intestinal microbiota following gastrointestinal stomas. This topic in particular looks at cases of stomas that need enteral feeding.

In the second section, "Stomas Prevention," there are two chapters. The chapter "Full Colonoscopy in Patients under 50 Years Old with Lower Gastrointestinal Bleeding" shows a clinical problem of great social impact: early diagnosis of colonic neoplasm from non-specific signs of gastrointestinal bleeding. This topic looks at the role of full colonoscopy compared with sigmoidoscopy and the usefulness of early diagnosis to prevent the risk of ostomy in the therapeutic program of colorectal cancer. The chapter "Radioimaging Diagnosis of Vaterian Ampulloma: Technique, Semiology, and Differential Diagnosis - Review" shows the complex diagnostic problem of perivaterian pathologies. Correct diagnosis allows the appropriate therapeutic choice to be made and reduces the risk of complications and intestinal stomas.

Vincenzo Neri
University of Foggia,
Italy

Section 1

Stoma Care

Chapter 1

Introductory Chapter: Role of Colostomy in the Colorectal Pathologies

Vincenzo Neri

1. Introduction

Gastrointestinal stomas can be performed during the surgical treatment of various colorectal diseases. The therapeutic indications of colostomy are the decompression in the treatment of intestinal obstruction or the need of definitive or temporary exclusion of intestinal transit.

2. Functional and anatomical characteristics of colostomy

The first subdivision is between temporary and definitive colostomy; this distinction is based on the therapeutic perspective. Following anatomical criterion, the stomas can be divided as terminal and parietal. The parietal colostomies encompass cecostomy and loop colostomy. They are usually temporary, and fecal diversion is often partial; their site can be right iliac fossa (cecostomy) or left iliac fossa (sigmoidostomy) and right paraumbilical site (transverse colonoscopy). Loop colostomy can be stabilized by a stick. Cecostomy usually is completed by the self-retained catheter fixed by the purse-string suture. Technical simplicity and rapid accomplishment are the characteristics of cecostomy. In the past, the parietal colostomies, as transverse colostomy, have been employed with the aim to prevent the leakage or dehiscence of the colorectal anastomosis, but now this role has been denied. In summary cecostomy may be indicated as a means of gas decompression in colonic obstruction, and transverse colostomy can instead ensure fecal diversion which is generally partial. End colostomy allows total fecal diversion. This can be employed in case of resection of diseased segment of the colon, and the immediate, contextual anastomosis is judged to be uncertain and not indicated. End colostomy is recommended rather than loop colostomy as permanent ostomy. In some conditions, such as Hartmann's procedure, there is also the distal end of the colon that can be treated as mucus fistula.

3. Indications for colostomy

The purpose of colostomy should be evaluated based on some reflections: clinical frame, functional aim, and temporal perspective of the procedure. The indications for colostomy can occur in the elective or urgent clinical conditions. The elective situation provides the bowel preparation; the patients may be submitted to the surgical procedure in the best general conditions. It will be also possible to choose the correct site on the abdominal wall of ostomy. Some clinical conditions that require elective temporary colostomy are the treatment of rectovaginal and rectovesical fistula and inflammatory perineal disease; temporary colostomy usually is required for the protection of insecure low colorectal anastomosis. More frequently colostomy in the emergent clinical conditions is performed. In the first line are the traumatic lesions of the colon such as penetrating injuries, sometimes inserted in the very complex abdominal trauma. Obstruction of the large bowel and colonic perforation are in some cases indication for emergency colostomy. The functional purpose of colostomy is the fecal diversion or anal substitution. The therapeutic indications that require fecal diversion are numerous: discharge of intestinal obstruction is the more frequent clinical condition that can be treated with ostomy, to prevent possible contamination from rectal lesions or the management of rectal disease as high rectal fistula, rectovaginal fistula, etc. The temporal perspective of colostomy allows the distinction between the temporary and permanent one. First of all, permanent colostomy is indicated if the location of malignancy requires the abdominal perineal resection. Severe anatomical damage of the anal sphincter occurs in the complex ischiorectal abscess, Fournier's gangrene, lymphogranuloma venereum, and other severe inflammatory diseases that involve the perineum. Temporary colostomy has numerous indications as reported above.

4. General considerations of surgical techniques

The most important considerations concern the kind and the site of pathological involvement of the colon, the presence of possible complications, the anatomical mobility of each colonic segments, and the problems related to the closure of temporary colostomy. Colostomy is usually performed on the mobile sections of the colon: cecum or transverse or sigmoid colon. The site of the colostomy on the abdominal wall should be not close to bone saliences as costal edge of the torax, anterior superior iliac spine because the difficult to put on the colostomy appliance. Generally transverse colostomy is placed between the umbilicus and VIII rib and sigmoid colostomy between the umbilicus and anterior superior iliac spine. It is always preferable that the specific skin incision is made for colostomy; it is not recommended that colostomy passes through laparotomy. The position of colostomy along the colon is significant, because proximal ostomy, as cecostomy, causes hydroelectrolytic loss and irritation and ulceration of the skin around; but the pathologies affect this choice.

5. Colostomy morbidity

There are specific complications of colostomy that can be subdivided as early and late. The early complications occur during the immediate postoperative phase and encompass ostomy necrosis, retraction, peristomal infection, wound breaking open, skin irritation, blockage of colostomy, and intestinal obstruction [1]. The late complications include ostomy stenosis, prolapse mucous or total, parastomal hernia, poor stoma siting, and mucocutaneous separation. The global incidence of colostomy complications shows a wide range from 6 to 59% [2]. This wide variation should be due to the confusing definition of ostomy complications; and some of these would be out the medical competence but linked to the difficult adaptation of the patient to new condition. However also other studies recently reported in the literature confirmed the high incidence and the wide variation of ostomy morbidity with the range between 10 and 82% [3]. There are in this section various risk factors. The operation-related risks as the emergency conditions play the remarkable role rather than elective indications of the procedure and the patient-related risk as the age, obesity and general conditions. Finally there are the disease-specific risk: ulcerative rectocolitis, Crohn disease, and ischemic colitis have more frequent colostomy complications. Alteration of vascular supply is a fearsome complication which can occur within 48–72 hours from the surgery. The vascular damage may be localized to the external, superficial section of the stoma or concerns the deep portion below the abdominal wall. The incidence of the superficial necrosis ranges between 2 and 20%; less frequent is the deep necrosis with the incidence of 0.37–3% [4]. The vascular damage is due to the excessive traction, torsion of the colic stump, or its excessive trimming of the epiploic fat and the mesentery. Very important in the prevention of the ischemic colostomy complication is the correct mobilization of the colonic segment which has to reach easily the skin site of the stoma. The superficial vascular compromission can be controlled and followed awaiting the resolution; if the ischemic evidence extends deeper, it is mandatory for the surgical revision to perform new colostomy. The stoma retraction generally is due to incomplete mobilization of the colon. The retraction is more frequent among the stoma complications; its incidence ranges between 30 and 40% [5]. This complication can occur early, in most cases for incorrect skin fixation, in particular in the obese patients; in this case, the dehiscence of mucocutaneous junction with site contamination is feared. It is also possible that the retraction develops late in the postoperative period, because of the patient's mobilization and deambulation. In some cases local revision can be attempted, but the success of this maneuver is unlikely because the retraction is usually due to incomplete colonic mobilization. Therefore the correction of colostomy retraction requires the new surgical procedure. Stoma stenosis can develop at the skin or fascial level; it is frequently caused by mucocutaneous dehiscence, peristomal contaminations, and suppurations with fibrosis. Fascial level stenosis may cause intestinal obstruction that should be treated by surgical procedure; the incomplete and superficial stenosis can be treated with conservative therapy and dilation procedures. Stomal prolapse is often a late complication, The incidence shows a wide range from 2 to 20% [6]. The prolapse can develop as simple mucosal prolapse or as a complete prolapse of all colonic wall. Loop colostomies are more frequently subject to complication than the end stomas. The causes of the prolapse are the excessive mobilization of the colon without the fixation of the mesentery and colon at fascial edge and finally can be also involved in the increase of the intra-abdominal pressure. Sometimes the stomal prolapse is voluminous and reducible. This is not a surgical emergency, but repeated reduction maneuvers are not recommended, and the complete surgical treatment should be performed. Parastomal hernia, incisional hernia, is unusual in the early postoperative period but becomes more frequently late, reaching the incidence of 15–40% [7]. The risk factors for the development of parastomal hernia are the large opening performed in the abdominal wall and the thin thickness of the abdominal wall. Such as for other abdominal wall hernias, all actions that increase the intra-abdominal pressure are important. In the parastomal hernia, it is possible that the common complications of hernias, as strangulation, irreducibility, and incarceration, require urgent surgical treatment. The therapeutic approach includes local primary repair, mesh repair, and relocation of the stoma. The simple repair of the parietal defect is followed by high recurrence rates which oscillate between 46% and 100%. These results are discouraging. The relocation of the stoma is usually performed in association with the parietal defect repair. This procedure provides better results, but the recurrence rates remains rather high (20–40%) [8]. The mesh repair of parastomal hernia with the stoma relocation, employing numerous technical details, has produced better results, reducing the incidence of recurrence to an acceptable level: 7–17% [9]. After some debatable suggestions to prevent parastomal hernia, as reduction of the size of trephination, passage of the colon through the rectus abdominis, and extraperitoneal passage of the colon, there is the current proposal of the use of prophylactic mesh added into primary operation to prevent parastomal hernia [10].

6. Colostomy closure

The technique of colostomy closure is dependent on the type of colostomy which was employed: loop, end, or minor modifications of these are the methods. The pathology and clinical situations encountered usually recommend which type of colostomy should be performed. Closure of loop colostomy can be a simple procedure but, in some cases, can be rather difficult based on the degree of inflammation, the presence of fibrosis, or scarring. The contentious technical features about loop closure encompass simple closure as alternative of resection and anastomosis, intra- versus extraperitoneal closure, and finally the use of peritoneal drainage. Closure of an end colostomy with Hartmann's procedure can be commonly more difficult than simple colostomy closure and sometimes may occur the postoperative complications. Closure of end colostomy and mucous fistula has been traditionally performed with a laparotomy, dissection, and release of both ostomies and end-to-end anastomosis.

Author details

Vincenzo Neri
University of Foggia, Italy

*Address all correspondence to: vincenzo.neri@unifg.it

References

[1] Kwiatt M, Kawata M. Avoidance and management of stoma complications. Clinics in Colon and Rectal Surgery. 2013;**26**:112-121

[2] Ratliff CR, Donovan AM. Frequency of peristomal complications. Ostomy/Wound Management. 2001;**47**:26-29

[3] Duchesne JC, Wang YZ, Weinstraub SL, et al. Stoma complications: A multivariate analysis. The American Surgeon. 2002;**68**:961-966

[4] Formijne HA, Draaisma WA, Roskott AM, et al. Early complications after stoma formation: A prospective cohort study in 100 patients with 1 year followup. International Journal of Colorectal Disease. 2012;**27**:1095-1099

[5] Nastro P, Knowles CH, Mc Grath A, et al. Complications of intestinal stomas. The British Journal of Surgery. 2010;**97**:1885-1889

[6] Harris DA, Egbeare D, Jones S, et al. Complications and mortality following stoma formation. Annals of the Royal College of Surgeons of England. 2005;**87**:427-431

[7] Rondelli F, Reboldi P, Rulli A, et al. Loop ileostomy versus loop colostomy for fecal diversion after colorectal or coloanal anastomosis: A meta-analysis. International Journal of Colorectal Disease. 2009;**24**:479-488

[8] Israelsson LA. Parastomal hernias. The Surgical Clinics of North America. 2008;**88**:113-125

[9] Riansuwan W, Hull TL, Millan MM, et al. Surgery of recurrent parastomal hernia: Direct repair or relocation? Colorectal Disease. 2010;**12**:681-686

[10] Hansson BM, Slater NJ, van der Velden, et al. Surgical techniques for parastomal hernia repair: A systematic review of the literature. Annals of Surgery. 2012;**255**:685-695

Chapter 2

Stoma Revision on the Flaps in Cases of Abdominal Wall Defect with Digestive Tract Rupture

Masaki Fujioka

Abstract

Several surgical methods are performed for the reconstruction of abdominal wall defects after abdominoperineal resection, involving re-suture and free skin grafting. In the complex surgical cases with large abdominal wall defects, the treatment of intestinal fistula and wound infection is challenging. In many cases, they also have had the problems of the control and reposition of a stoma, which has been already present due to the previous unsuccessful surgical procedures. Especially, the case of larger abdominal wall defects with intestinal fistulation, which drains digestive juice into the wound, requires repairing the abdominal wall while fashioning a stoma. This is because a ruptured digestive tract causes infection and inflammation that results in adhesion of the digestive tract, which limits the mobility of both the abdominal wall and bowel. The only method to solve this complex problem is abdominal wall reconstruction with a large vascularized flap and creation of a new stoma on it to separate the wound from drained digestive juice. We present several cases of a large abdominal wall defect, which was reconstructed successfully. Especially, surgical methods using free and perforator flaps are highlighted. These are optimal methods to reconstruct severe abdominal wall defects that involve complications.

Keywords: stoma, flap, abdominal wall defect, digestive tract rupture, surgical site infection

1. Introduction

Intestinal stomas are surgically created openings of either the small or large bowel into the anterior abdominal wall. They are often necessary to prevent devastating complications or save a patient's life [1]. Permanent stomas are required when altered anatomy prohibits the re-establishment of gastrointestinal continuity or the risks of undergoing another surgery are prohibitive due to the patient's poor condition. A well-made stoma will have the largest impact on the patient's long-term quality of life.

The principles of stoma creation are typically the same: the opening is created in the abdominal wall, a segment of the bowel is delivered through the external and internal oblique and transversus muscles, and the bowel is opened and secured to the skin [1]. Thus, successful stoma creation requires a healthy abdominal wall and a well-vascularized, tension-free segment of bowel [1, 2].

However, patients who have undergone prior abdominal surgery and developed bowel inflammation and adhesion present with problems, if they require emergent ileostomy for infection or fistulization. Especially, when an abdominal surgical site infection associated with abdominal wall defect develops, fashioning an intestinal stoma is very challenging [3, 4].

In these cases, reconstruction of a wall defect after abdominoperineal resection is very demanding with regard to the functional outcome. Several surgical methods have been performed involving re-suture, free skin grafting, and local flaps, which can be useful when the defect is relatively small [4]. However, larger abdominal wall defects usually require large flaps [5–7]. If the bilateral abdominal skin was not damaged by previous surgical procedures, abdominal defect may be reconstructed using a large pedicled flap. On the other hand, in the case of larger defects with further complications, such as an antecedent formation of a colostomy or iliac conduit, the free flap transfer is required, because local flaps around the wound cannot be harvested due to the damages of the abdominal skin.

The aim of this article is to describe techniques of stoma creation on the flaps in cases of postoperative fascial necrosis with internal bowel fistulae causing continuous peritoneal contamination. Especially, surgical methods for the two major types of the complications: abdominal wall defect with wound infection "with and without previous stoma" using free and perforator flaps are especially highlighted.

2. Case presentations of abdominal wall defect with wound infection with and without the previous stoma

2.1 Case1. Abdominal reconstruction with a free latissimus dorsi musclocutaneous flap for the patient with previous stoma

A 38-year-old female originally had squamous cell carcinoma of the cervix uteri and had undergone radical hysterectomy and oophorectomy followed by postoperative chemotherapy and radiotherapy. After a disease-free period of 13 years, cervical cancer recurred, and she underwent pelvic exenteration including the bladder, rectum, sigmoid colon, and vagina. The end colostomy and ileal conduit were fashioned. However, her postoperative course was complicated by small bowel necrosis, which required another laparotomy to remove it. The mid-abdominal wound developed dehiscence. The pelvic cavity, which extended from the pubic symphysis to the coccyx internally and communicated with the perineal defect measuring 8 × 6 cm, was packed with saline-soaked gauze dressing every day. The remaining bowel and omentum were adherent at the center of the abdominal cavity, possibly due to the previous radiation (**Figures 1–3**). Furthermore, the adhered colon developed necrosis, which drained stools into the pelvic cavity, resulting in chronic peritonitis (**Figures 4** and **5**). Surgery was planned so that the empty pelvic cavity could be filled with a large vascularized muscle to prevent chronic peritonitis and create a new stoma for the ruptured colon to separate the pelvic cavity from drained stools (**Figure 6**). At first, the abdominal full-thickness defect combined with its communication with the pelvic cavity was de-epithelialized and curetted carefully. The patient was then placed in a right lateral decubitus position, and a left combined serratus anterior and latissimus dorsi musclocutaneous flaps with a 25 × 7-cm elliptical skin island, both of which were based on the thoracodorsal vessels, was harvested in the standard manner (**Figure 7**).

Following primary closure of the donor defect, these muscle flaps were inserted into the pelvic cavity. Then, the thoracodorsal artery was connected by end-to-end anastomosis with a branch of the profunda femoris artery, and two thoracodorsal veins were connected by end-to-end anastomosis with the branches of the venae

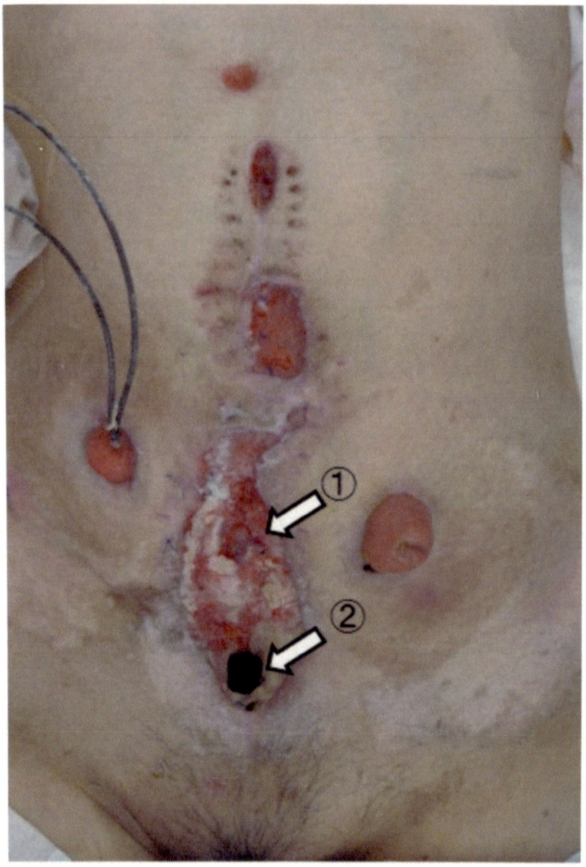

Figure 1.
A view of the abdominal wound, demonstrating the ruptured colon at the center of the abdominal cavity (1), and the fistula penetrating the pelvic cavity (2).

comitantes of this profunda femoris (**Figure 8**). Finally, a skin paddle was applied to cover the abdominal fistula, and a new colon stoma was fashioned through the slit made in the skin flap (**Figures 9** and **10**).

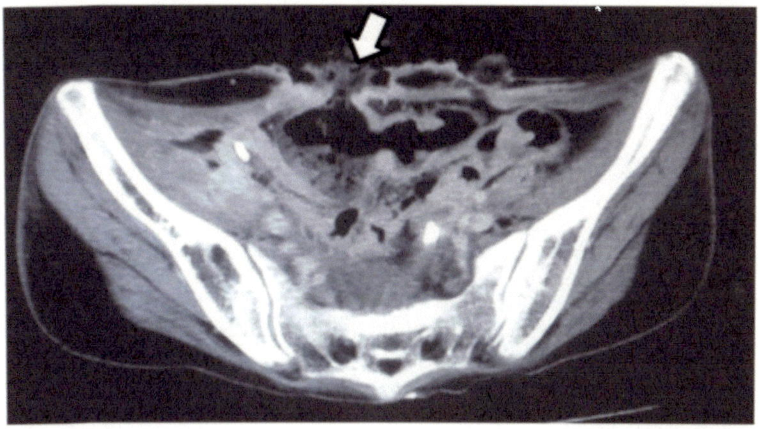

Figure 2.
Computed tomography scan image demonstrating a necrotic colon (arrow).

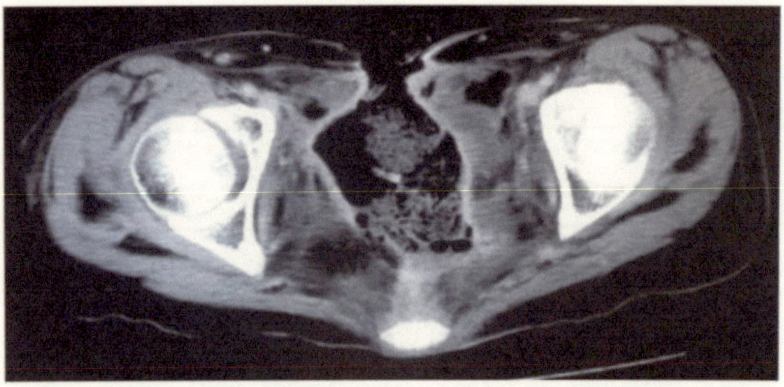

Figure 3.
Computed tomography scan image demonstrating the pelvic cavity, which extended from the pubic symphysis to coccyx internally.

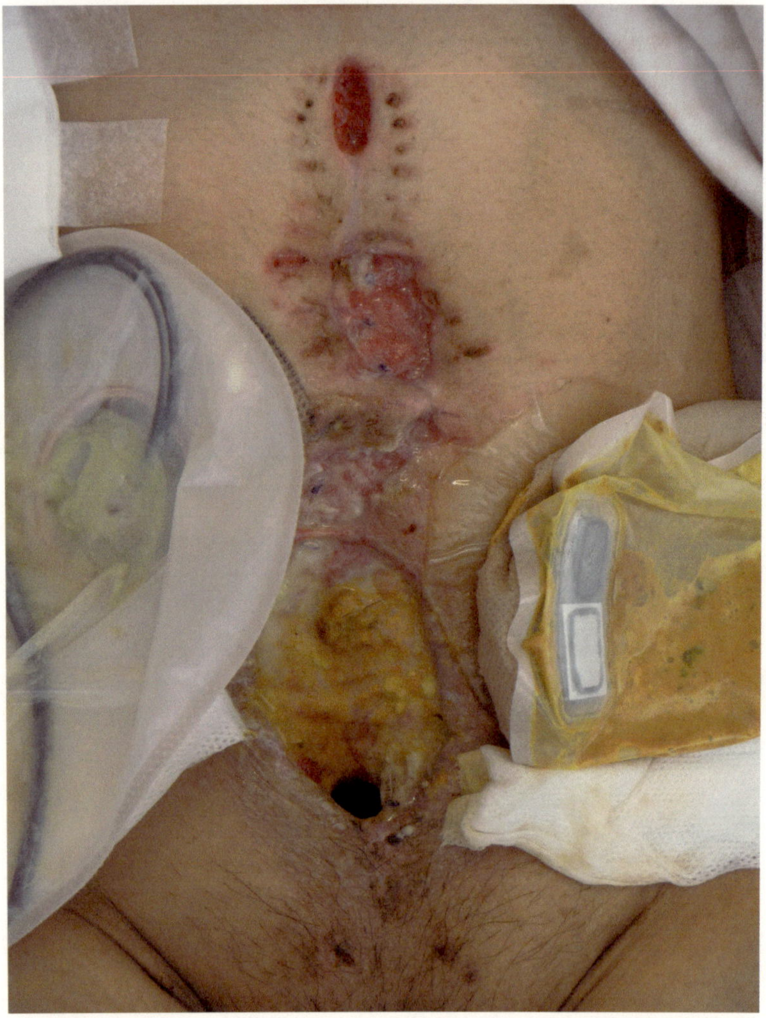

Figure 4.
A view of the abdominal wound, demonstrating that the ruptured colon drained stools into the pelvic cavity, resulting in chronic peritonitis.

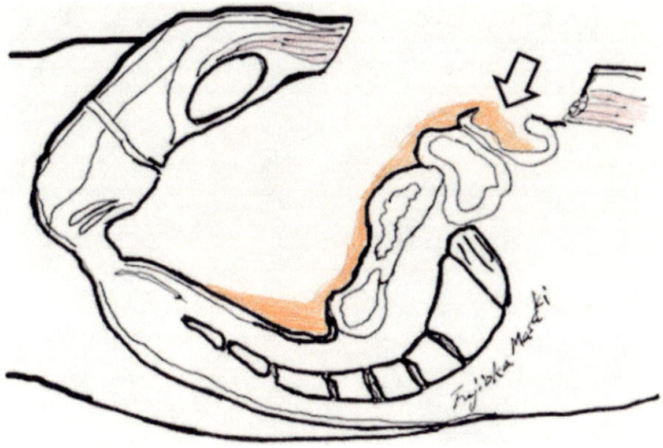

Figure 5.
Illustration of the sagittal section demonstrating the ruptured colon (arrow) and fistula in the pelvic cavity.

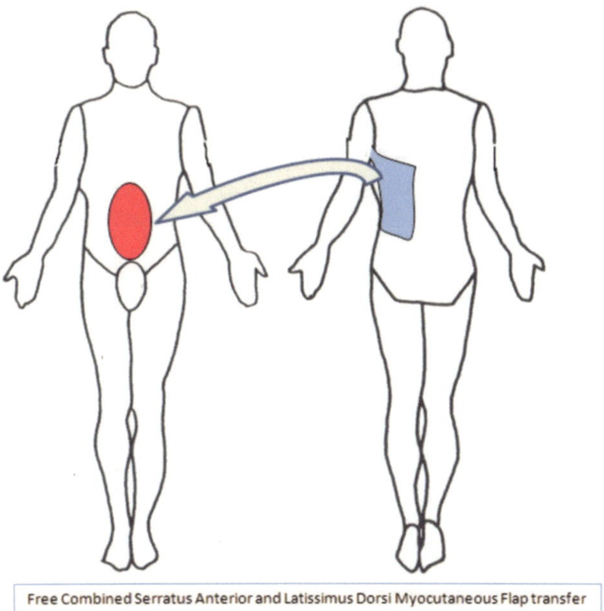

Figure 6.
Schematic illustration of the surgical procedure of free combined serratus anterior and latissimus dorsi musclocutaneous flaps transfer.

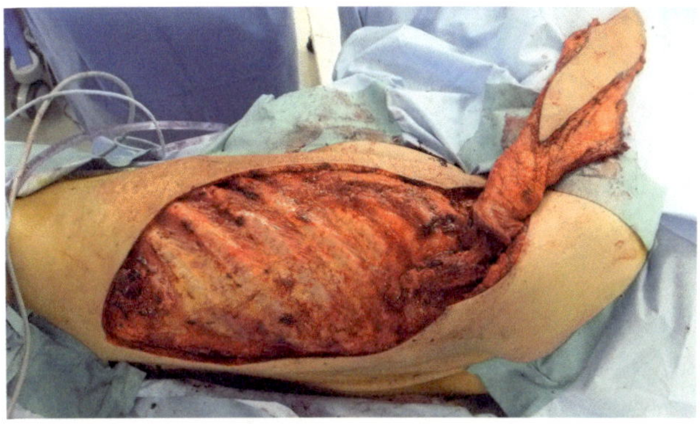

Figure 7.
Intraoperative view showing a left combined serratus anterior and latissimus dorsi musclocutaneous flaps with a skin island.

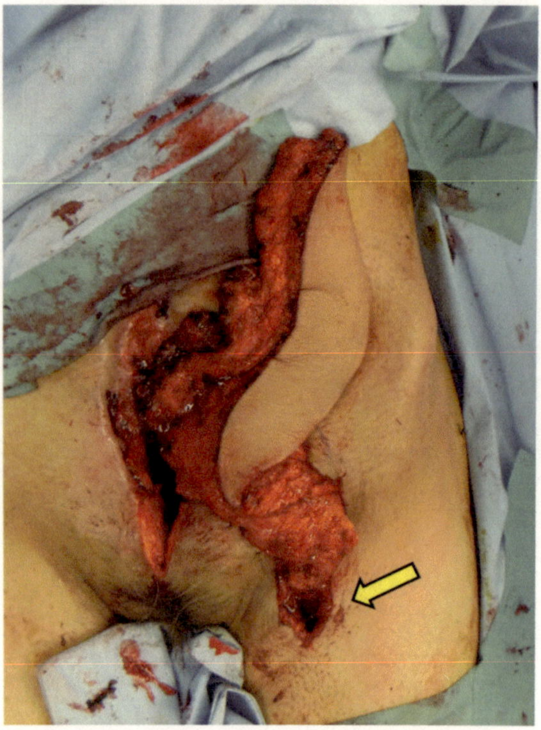

Figure 8.
Intraoperative view showing the muscle flaps inserted into the pelvic cavity and the thoracodorsal vessels connected with a branch of the deep vessels of the thigh (arrow).

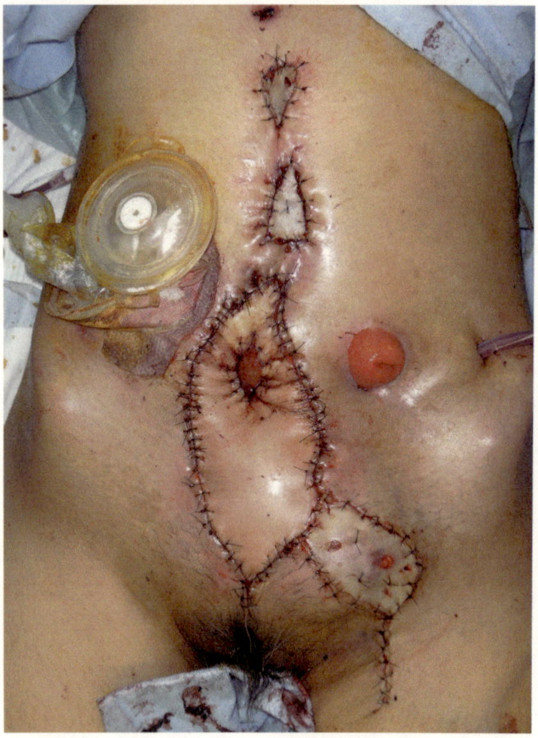

Figure 9.
Intraoperative view showing a skin paddle applied to cover the abdominal fistula and a new colon stoma fashioned through the slit made in the skin flap.

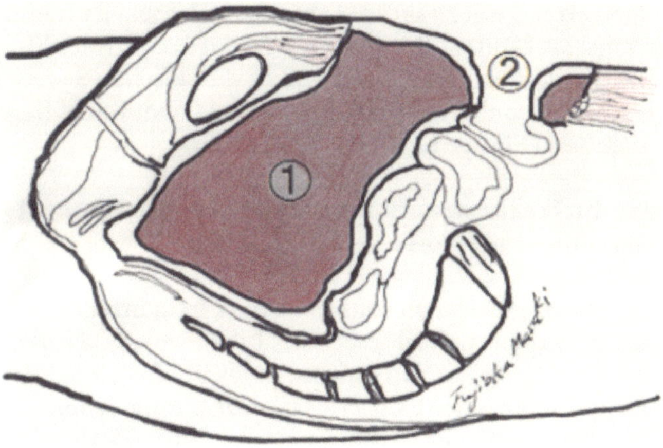

Figure 10.
Illustration of a sagittal section demonstrating the pelvic cavity filled with the muscle (1) and a new colon stoma fashioned in the skin flap (2).

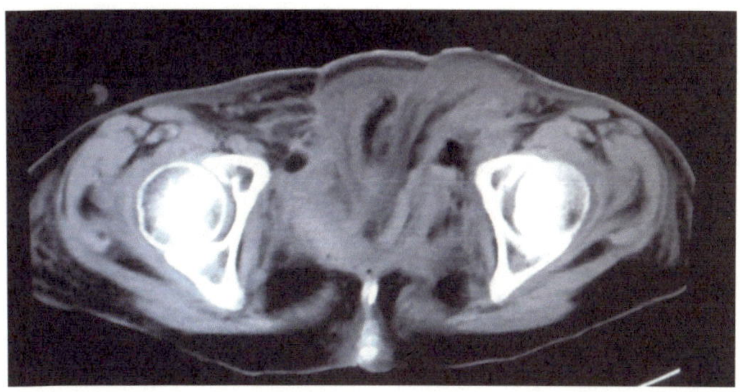

Figure 11.
Computed tomography scan image taken after 2 weeks, showing the pelvic cavity filled with the transported muscle.

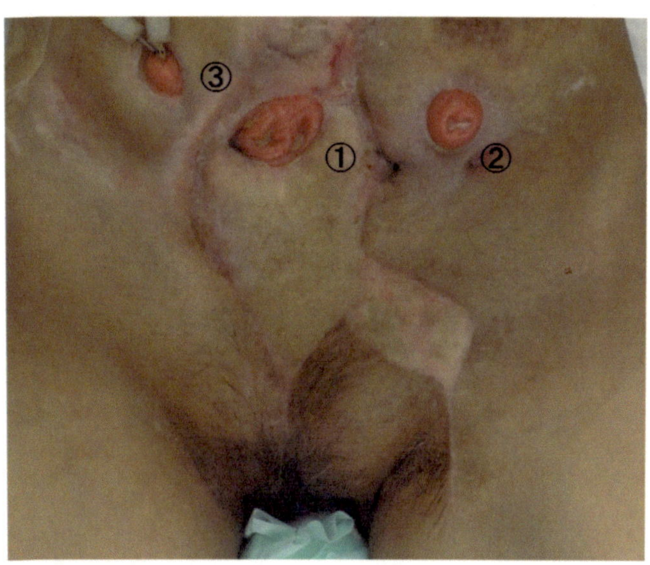

Figure 12.
A view of the abdominal wall 3 months after surgery revealed favorable coverage of the wound and a new colon stoma fashioned on the flap (1). It also showed a conventional stoma (2) and conventional urinary stoma (3).

A CT scan taken after 2 weeks showed that the pelvic cavity had been filled with the transported muscles (**Figure 11**). She underwent excess free skin grafting due to partial necrosis developing at the distal end of the skin flap 3 weeks later. Three months later, the patient could walk in the absence of abdominal hernia formation and relapse of infection (**Figure 12**).

2.2 Case 2. Abdominal reconstruction with pedicled perforator flaps for the patient without previous stoma

A 66-year-old male originally had squamous cell carcinoma of the lower esophagus (Stage III) and had undergone radical resection of the esophageal cancer followed by reconstruction using free jejunum flap transfer. However, his postoperative course was complicated by peritonitis due to a perforation of the duodenum on the next day, which required another emergency laparotomy to cleanse and close the duodenal fistula. The mid-abdominal wound, which extended from the pubic symphysis to the processus xiphoideus, measuring 25 × 6 cm, developed infection and dehiscence 4 days after the primary surgery (**Figure 13**). Thus, the patient underwent debridement, and the wound was packed with saline-soaked gauze dressing every day. Furthermore, the exposed small intestine, which was adherent and fixed at the center of the abdominal wound, developed necrosis and drained digestive juice into the wound, resulting in a contaminated chronic ulcer 10 days after the primary surgery (**Figure 14**).

Reconstruction surgery was performed 20 days after the primary surgery, so that the open wound could be resurfaced with a large vascularized flap to prevent chronic contamination and create a new ileostoma for the ruptured ileum to separate the wound from drained digestive juice. The abdominal full-thickness defect was curetted carefully, and two triangular fasciocutaneous flaps of 25 × 7 cm, both of which were based on the perforator vessels of the lower abdominal artery, were harvested bilaterally (**Figure 15**).

Following primary closure of the donor sites, these perforator flaps were transferred medially to resurface the exposed small intestine. The ruptured ileum was encircled by these two flaps, and the mucosa of the small intestine was sutured to the skin of the flaps; consequently, an ileostoma was fashioned between the skin flaps (**Figure 16**). The remaining upper and lower abdominal wounds were resurfaced using free skin grafting.

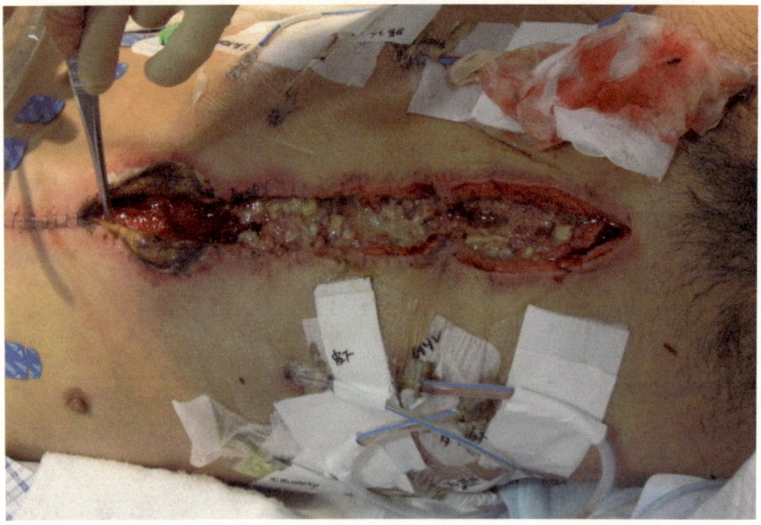

Figure 13.
A view of the abdominal wound, demonstrating infection and dehiscence.

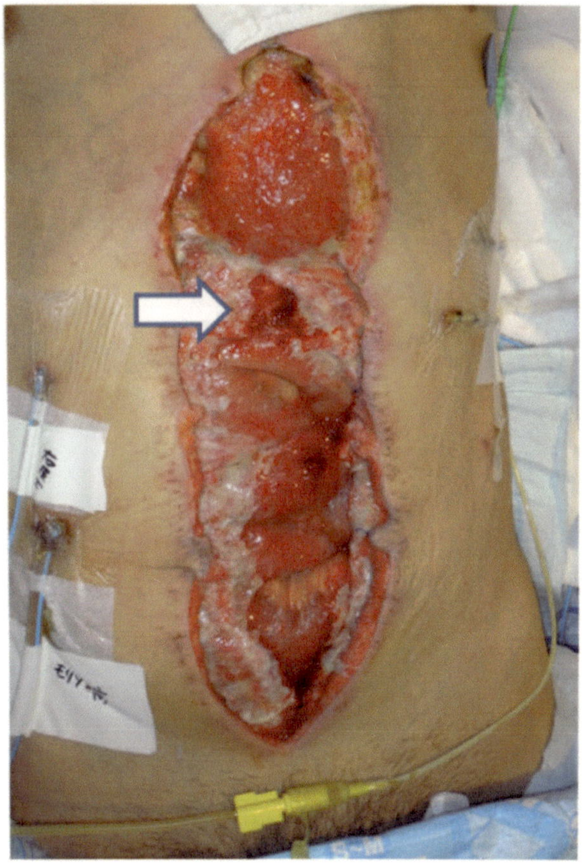

Figure 14.
A view of the abdominal wound after debridement, demonstrating the exposed small intestine, which ruptured and developed a fistula (arrow).

Three months later, all abdominal wounds had resurfaced, and the draining digestive juice could be controlled using a stoma bag. The patient could walk in the absence of abdominal hernia formation and relapse of infection (**Figures 17** and **18**).

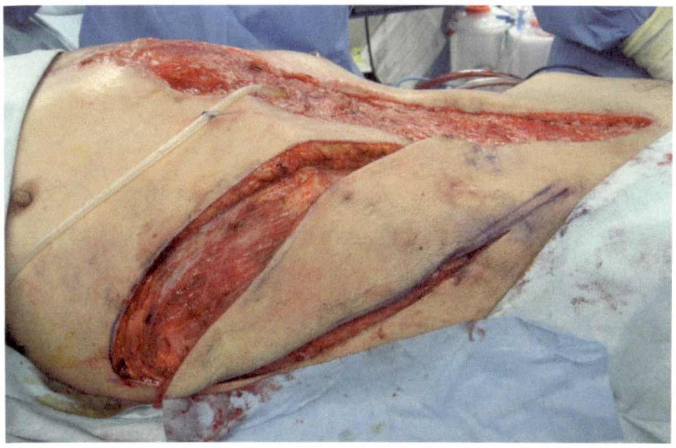

Figure 15.
A view of flap elevation, involving a triangular fasciocutaneous flap, fed by the perforator vessels of the lower abdominal artery.

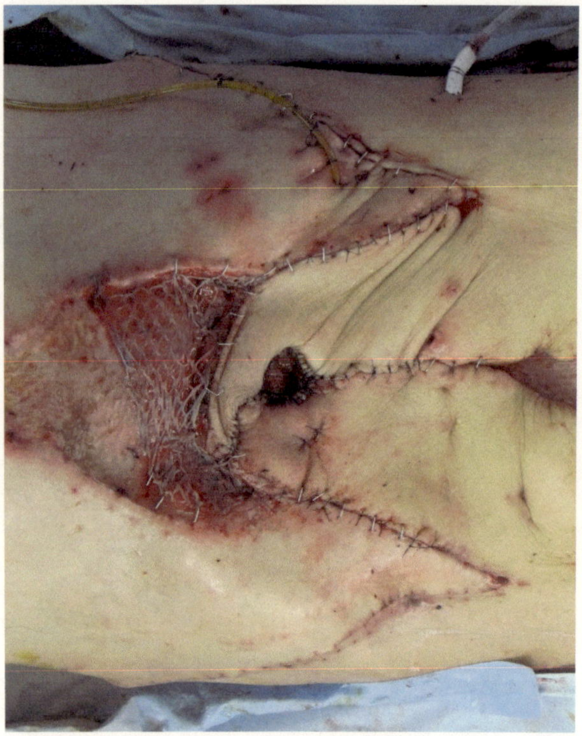

Figure 16.
A view of ileostoma creation; the ruptured ileum was encircled by two flaps.

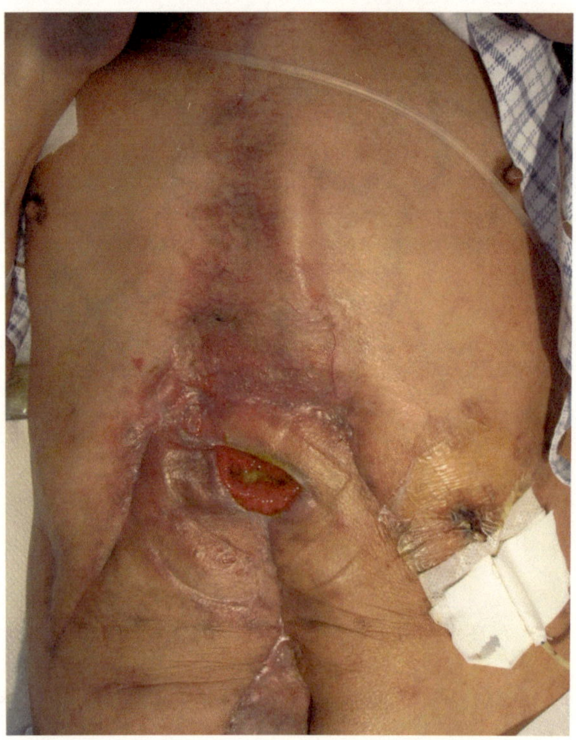

Figure 17.
A view of the abdominal wound 3 months after the surgery, showing that all abdominal wounds had resurfaced.

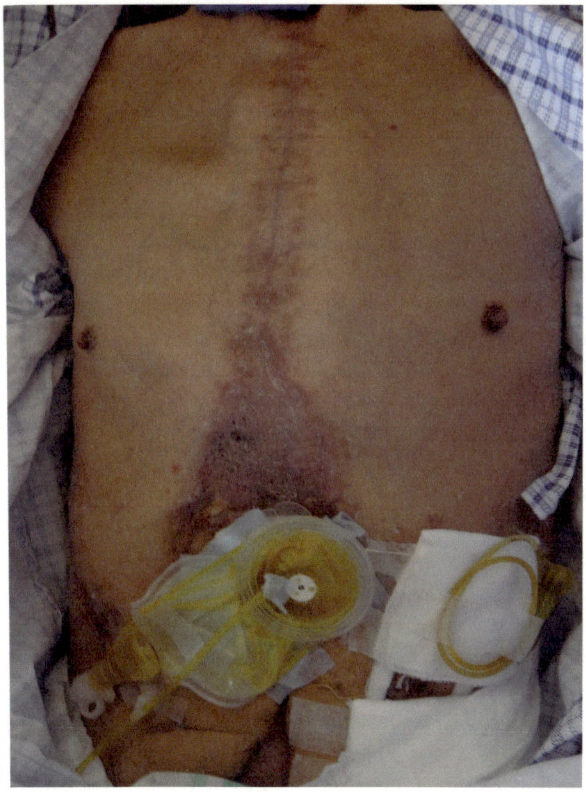

Figure 18.
The draining digestive juice could be controlled using a stoma bag.

3. Discursion

3.1 Management of complex abdominal wall wounds

Management of the patients with infected abdominal wounds associated with bowel fistulae is complicated, and the condition may prove fatal. Kendrick et al. reviewed 21 patients with severe postoperative soft tissue necrosis of the abdominal wall with and without associated intestinal fistulae and reported an overall survival rate of only 71% [8].

Regarding the treatment of an enterocutaneous fistula resulting from invasive bowel infection, en bloc resection of the involved bowel and enterocutaneous fistula tract with a healthy tissue margin while employing direct abdominal wall closure may be an ideal surgical treatment [9]. If the intestinal fistulation cannot be closed directly and end-to-end bowel anastomosis after ruptured intestine removal is not possible, the treatment for these patients becomes complicated, because debridement of contaminated soft tissue, abdominal wall reconstruction, and stoma fashioning are required at the same time [10].

In the procedure of fashioning a stoma, patients who have undergone prior complex abdominal operations present with difficulty due to an edematous and friable bowel and intra-abdominal adhesion, which decrease bowel mobilization. In these cases, the bowel is fixed on the adhesive mass of inflammation, making it difficult to deliver a well-vascularized, tension-free segment of bowel to the normal skin area and secure it through an adequate site of the abdominal wall [3, 11]. Furthermore, the inflammatory and exposed bowel caused by the wound dehiscence tends to develop ischemia and necrosis, which can result in intestinal rupture.

The drained digestive juice and stool from the fistulae spread and worsen the soft tissue infection. Ileostomy effluent, with an alkaline pH and containing active digestive enzymes, is discharged almost continuously and excoriates and digests unprotected skin if left exposed. A colostomy discharges feces, which can cause continuous contamination of wounds [12]. Many of these patients have lost substantial soft tissue to resurface the wound, due to prior enterectomy resulting in reduced compliance of the skin and abdominal wall caused by multiple operations, stomas, abscesses, and enterocutaneous fistulae [13].

The procedure for fashioning an ileostomy or colostomy is well established and straightforward in typical cases. However, problems such as intra-abdominal adhesions, bowel rupture with infection, and abdominal wall defect are difficult to manage [14]. In this context, the key point of managing these complex wounds is to create a stoma on the durable skin and separate the wound from the ileostomy effluent. To achieve this the area around the fistulae should be resurfaced with well-vascularized skin flaps.

3.2 Surgical reconstruction of the abdominal wall

Regarding abdominal wall reconstruction, several surgical methods include primary closure with and without artificial instruments, tissue expanders, component separation, and the use of local, regional, or free flaps [9]. Simultaneous reconstruction of the abdominal wall with prosthetic mesh is associated with a particularly high incidence of recurrent postoperative fistulation. Repair of contaminated abdominal wall defects with non-cross-linked biologic mesh and a component separation technique led to 36 of 80 patients (45%) developing wound infection [15]. Also, artificial mesh disturbs intestinal penetration though the abdominal wall [16]. Adaptations of artificial fascia are not adequate to resurface these contaminated wounds, because these non-vascularized substances are foreign bodies, which can aggravate infection [17–19]. Tissue expanders are used with the aim of expanding the skin around the wound [20]. They can provide the skin that can be used to cover large defects. However, this technique also requires the use of a foreign body in patients, which is a risk of infection, and there are space limitations caused by enterocutaneous fistulae, scar tissue, and stomas [2].

If the abdominal wall defect has a moderate size, but direct wound closure is impossible, abdominal repair with the component separation method, which is one of rectus abdominis muscle advancement flaps, is an alternative technique. This method can be accomplished without the need for artificial mesh, so it is also recommended from an infection control perspective (**Figure 19**) [21]. Separation of the muscle components of the abdominal wall allows mobilization of the rectus abdominal muscle, which enables each unit of the muscle to be sutured directly, and the stoma can be created through the reconstructed muscle. The external oblique muscle is bluntly dissected from the underlying internal oblique muscle, which should result in approximately 5 cm of advancement in the upper third of the abdomen, 10 cm in the mid-abdomen, and 3 cm in the lower third of the abdomen (**Figures 20–22**). This method is easy to perform without requiring the transposition of remote myocutaneous flaps or free tissue transfers [22, 23].

If wide and contaminated abdominal wounds cannot be closed directly, even with the component separation technique, pedicled or free flap transfer is required to resurface the wound [24, 25]. Kayano et al. compared 8 free anterolateral thigh (ALT) flaps and 12 pedicled ALT flaps for abdominal wall reconstruction to investigate their associated complications and clinical and demographic data and concluded that complication rates do not differ between free and pedicled ALT flaps. They suggested that the choice of flap depends on the size and location of the defect and the length of the vascular pedicle [26].

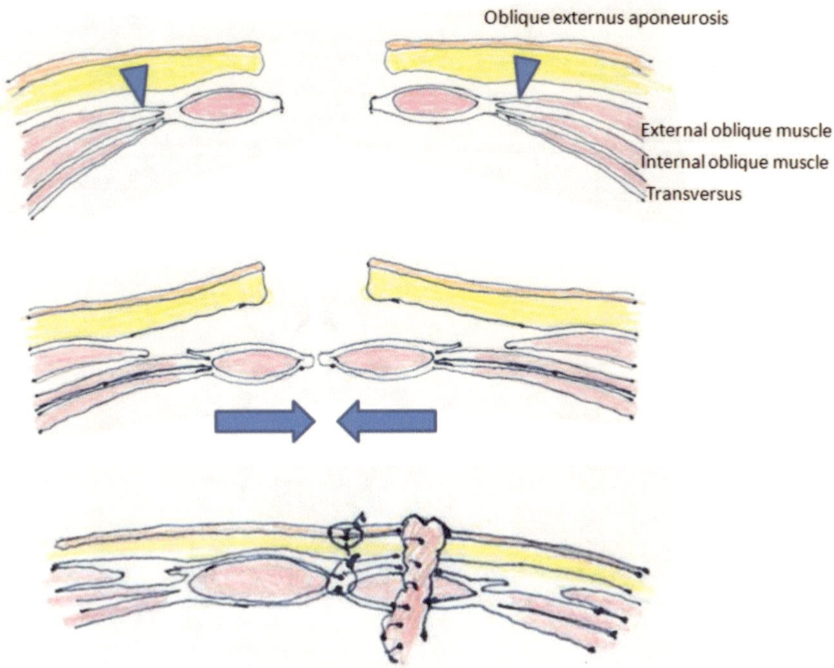

Figure 19.
Schematic illustration of abdominal wall repair with the component separation technique to enable primary fascial closure.

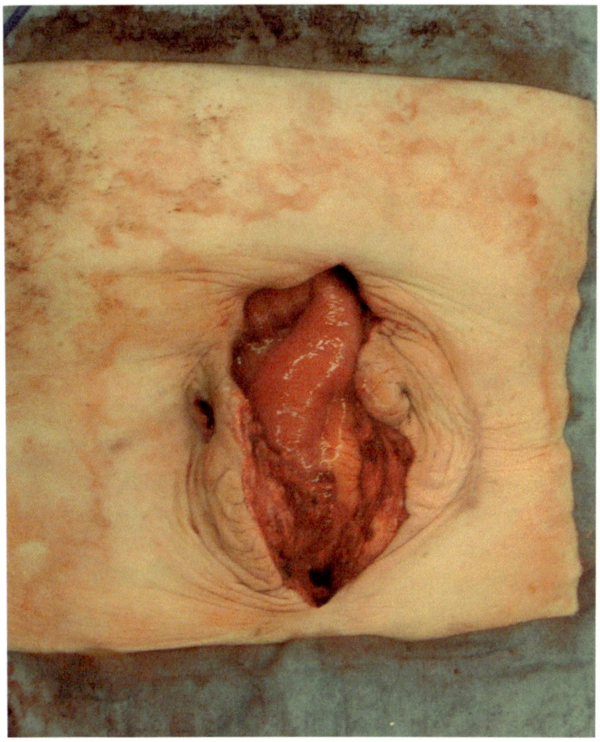

Figure 20.
Abdominal wall defect with a 7-cm width developed after debridement of contaminated skin and muscle.

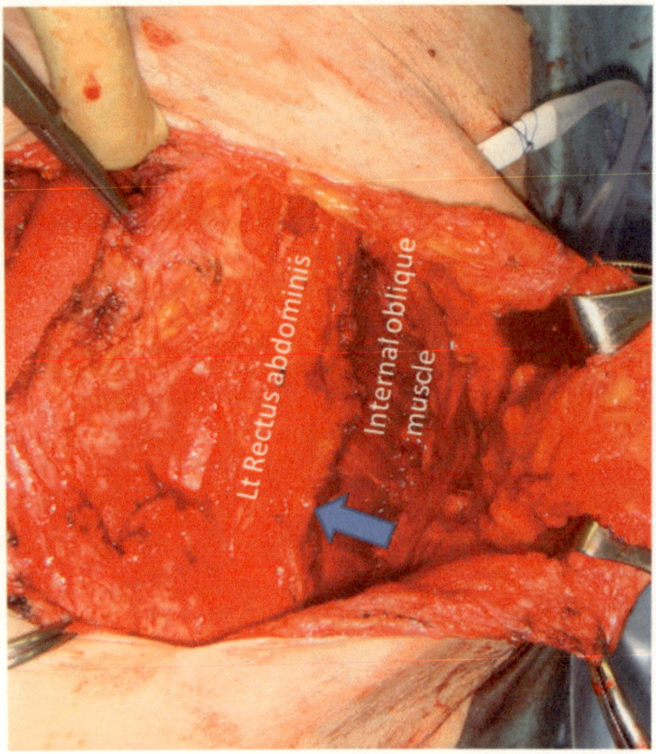

Figure 21.
The external oblique muscle was dissected from the underlying internal oblique muscle, which allowed rectus abdominal muscle advancement 4 cm median-ward (arrow).

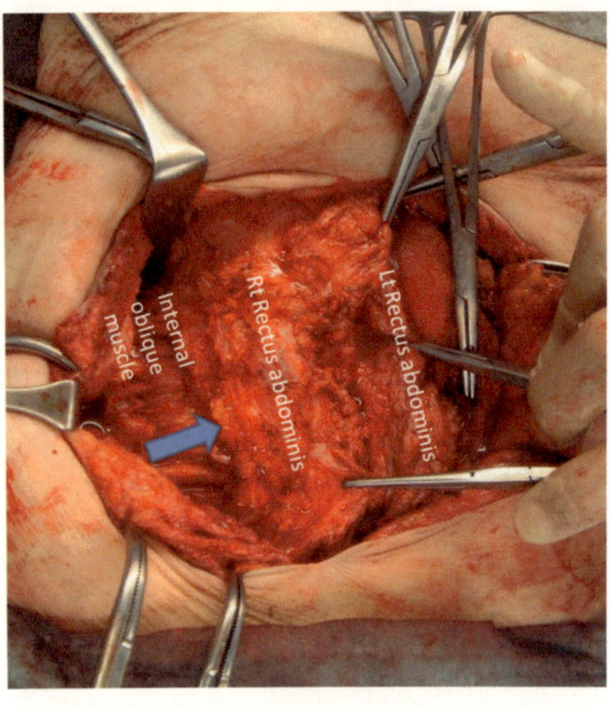

Figure 22.
Bilateral separation of the muscle components of the abdominal wall allows mobilization of the rectus abdominal muscle, enabling each unit of the muscle to be sutured directly.

Several case series revealed that a large flap is usually required for repair in the presence of larger defects with further complications, such as the formation of intestinal fistulae, and wound infection [5–7]. Reconstruction of a lower abdominal defect (below the umbilicus) can be achieved using pedicled ATL and tensor fascia lata fasciocutaneous (TFL) flaps. A retrospective study that analyzed 27 patients with abdominal wall defects concluded that both pedicled ATL and TFL fasciocutaneous flaps may be good options for the reconstruction of lower abdominal wall defects. A pedicled TFL fasciocutaneous flap has usually been utilized for lower abdominal defects (**Figures 23–26**) [27]. A pedicled ALT flap may be a better option for the reconstruction of a lower abdominal wall defect, and it is also available for whole abdominal wall defect restoration (**Figures 27–29**). This flap has the following advantages: it can be harvested as a musculocutaneous flap with the vastus lateralis muscle to fill a tissue defect, and the lack of a need for position change enables flap harvest [28, 29]. Regrettably, several case series showed that these useful flaps, which are harvested from the thigh, cannot reach the upper umbilical area, and the distal third of the TFL flap is at risk of necrosis unless a delaying procedure is used [5–7].

Consequently, free flap transfer has been traditionally chosen as the only suitable method to resurface a large upper abdominal defect [30]. A free musculocutaneous flap is supplied by large blood vessels that may promote the healing process in contaminated tissue [31]. This is because massive vascularized muscle transfer can be undertaken through the removal of contaminated tissue, and muscle flaps for dead-space obliteration and neovascularization are obligatory for successful management of such infected wounds [32, 33]. However, when performing free flap transfer around the contaminated area, identifying an acceptable recipient vessel is not always easy. Chronic inflammation in recipient vessels caused by infection and fibrosis may be one of the factors leading to thrombosis of an anastomosed vessel [34]. So, it is important to select a flap with a long pedicle, as a suitable recipient vessel may be distant from the wound. Abdominal muscle defects require synthetic materials or flaps for restoration to prevent hernias. The insertion of synthetic materials has been reserved for large defects of the abdominal wall, but they have demonstrated increased complication rates, especially in contaminated wounds [5, 27]. Therefore, a myocutaneous free flap is also desirable. The close continuity of the remaining rectus abdominis muscle after debridement and thick and bulky muscle in the transferred flap will prevent hernia formation [6].

Microsurgical free flap transfer may be one of the best options to repair soft tissue defects of the abdominal wall, as it can prevent a hernia and relapse of infection and supply a well-vascularized muscle and large durable skin paddle, which enable stoma fashioning on it [30].

Recently, anatomical understanding of the perforator and angiosomes has increased, allowing regional flaps to cover skin defects, providing an alternative to free flaps [35–37]. Perforator flaps are defined as flaps consisting of the skin and/or subcutaneous fat, with a blood supply from isolated perforating vessels of a stem artery [38]. This new concept highlights again that local flaps are a good option for covering a difficult area around a contaminated wound. An ideal flap is thought to be a good vascularized skin paddle with the same thickness and width as the wound and a single-stage operation [39]. The development of perforator flaps has increased the number of potential donor sites because a flap can be supplied by any musculocutaneous perforator, and donor-site morbidity can be reduced.

Perforator and fasciocutaneous rotation flaps avoid the sacrificing of the underlying muscle and are commonly used due to their advantages. Sameem M et al.

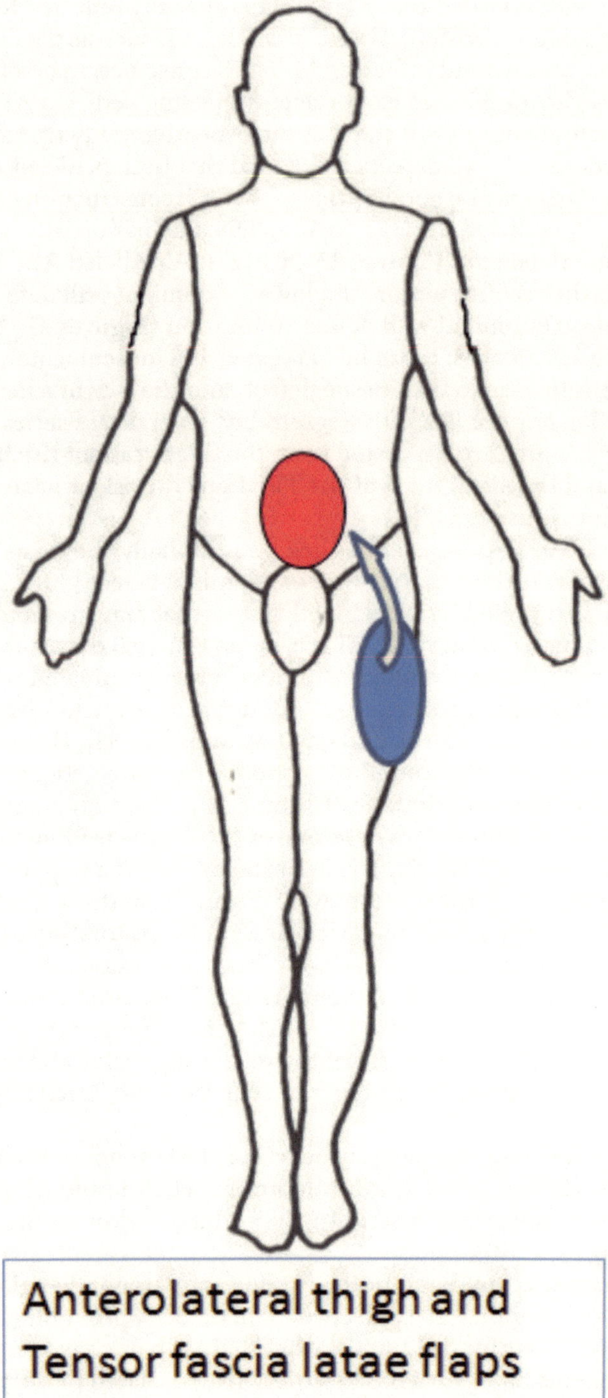

Figure 23.
Schematic illustration of lower abdominal wall repair using anterolateral thigh and tensor fascia lata flaps.

reviewed complications of musculocutaneous, fasciocutaneous, and perforator flaps for the treatment of pressure ulcers and revealed that there was no significant difference with regard to complication rates among these flaps [40]. However, comparing perforator and fasciocutaneous rotation flaps, application of the perforator

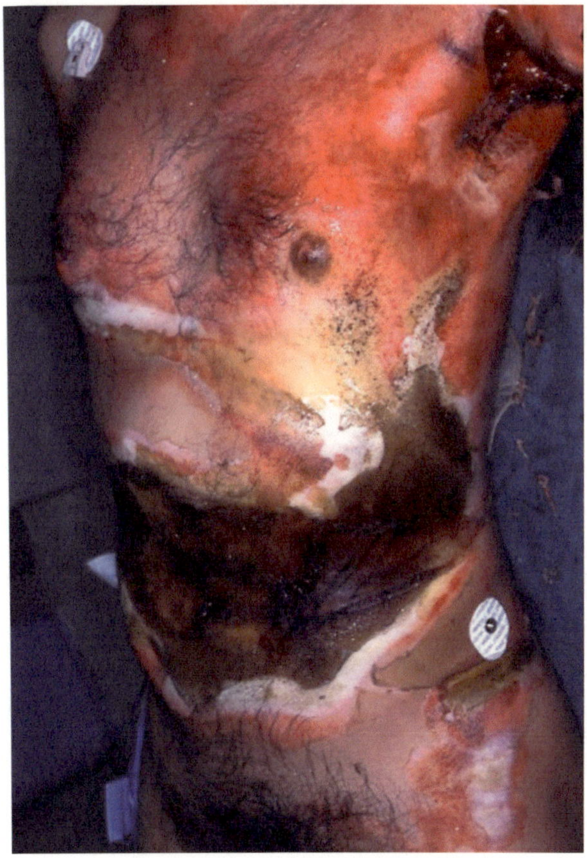

Figure 24.
A man sustained severe full-thickness abdominal burns due to contact with a large iron bowl (about 200°C) for 15 min, which was used for boiling sweet beans.

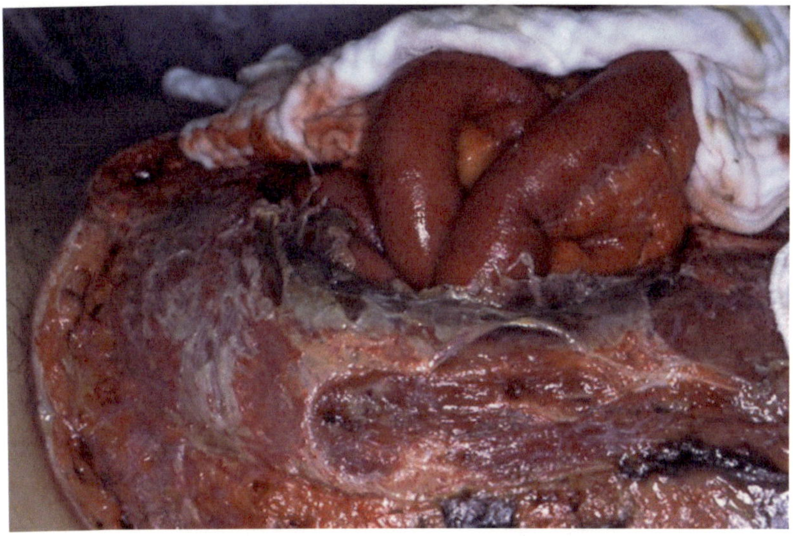

Figure 25.
The abdominal wall ruptured and the intestines were exposed due to the abdominal akin and muscle necrosis.

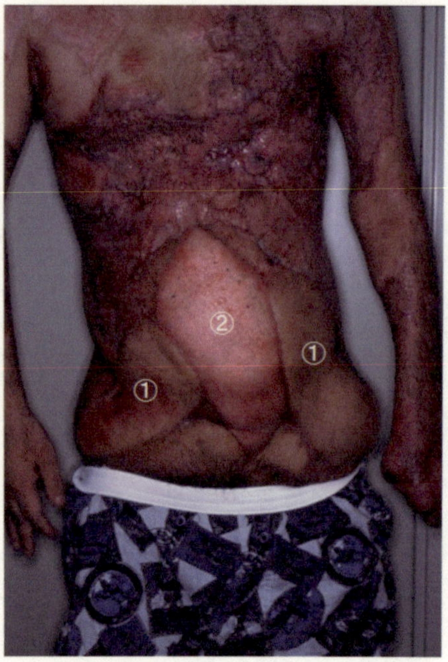

Figure 26.
View of the abdominal wall 9 months after reconstruction, using two pedicled TFL fasciocutaneous (1) and a free latissimus dorsi musclocutaneous (2) flaps.

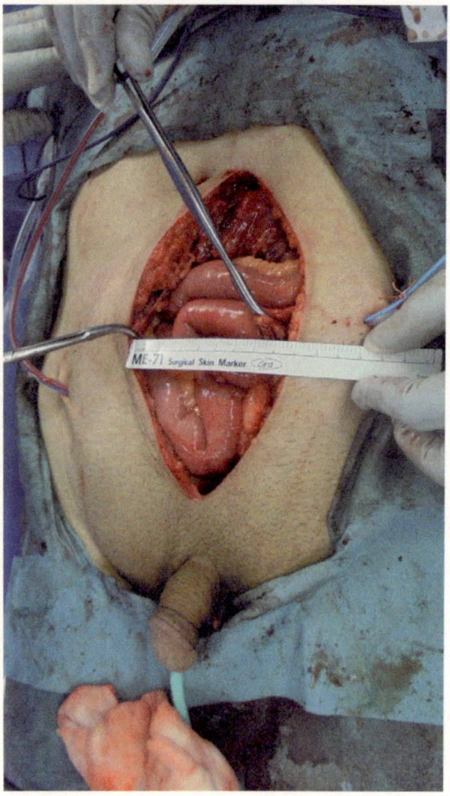

Figure 27.
Rectus abdominal muscle defect with a 9-cm width developed after debridement of contaminated muscle.

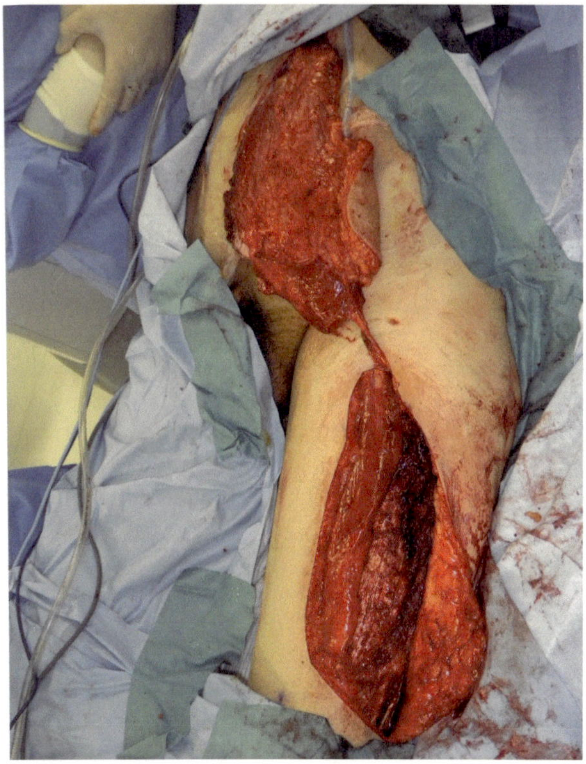

Figure 28.
A pedicled vastus lateralis-anterolateral thigh flap was elevated from the left thigh and transferred to the abdominal wall defect.

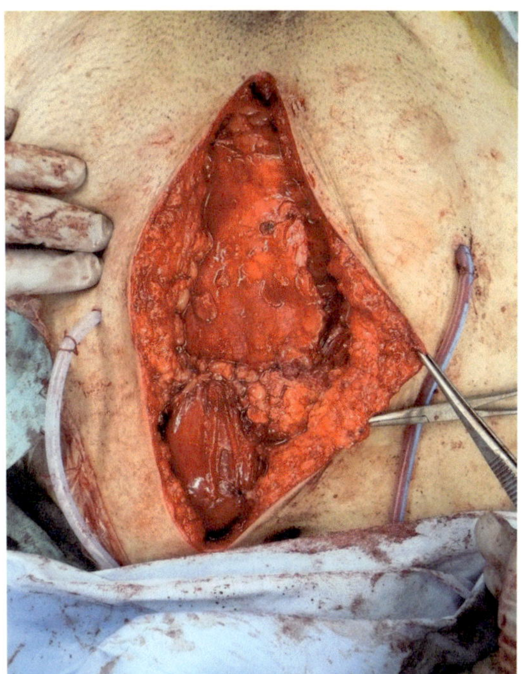

Figure 29.
The muscle flap was tunneled under the rectus femoris muscle and transferred to the muscle defect.

flap concept has many advantages. Parrett et al. revealed in a retrospective study that analyzed 290 flaps that blood circulation of the perforator flaps is supplied from isolated perforating vessels of a stem artery [38]. So, the most significant advantage of the perforator flap is that there is no need to sacrifice any main arteries, which means that there is minimal morbidity at the donor site [41, 42]. Also, microvascular anastomoses have the potential disadvantages that they require high-level surgical skill and prolong the operative period.

This new concept highlights again that local flaps could be a good option for the coverage of a difficult area of the upper abdomen, whose optimal reconstruction was previously thought to be possible with only free flap transfer.

Bilateral lower abdominal artery perforator flaps provide a well-vascularized skin paddle with an easy procedure, which does not require complicated microsurgical techniques. I believe that the use of this perforator flap is a good option to reconstruct large abdominal wall defects associated with many complications.

4. Conclusion

Reconstruction of a major abdominal wall defect in patients with a non-healing wound with infection due to continuous contamination from the ruptured ileum is challenging. The main problem is to separate the wound from draining digestive juice. A simple and the recommended method is stoma use, which requires a durable skin component in order to create a new stoma. To resolve these problems, flap transfer is required.

Conflict of interest

This manuscript has not benefited from any source of funding support or grants, and the author has no conflicting financial interest.

Author details

Masaki Fujioka[1,2]

1 Department of Plastic and Reconstructive Surgery, National Hospital Organization Nagasaki Medical Center, Ohmura, Nagasaki, Japan

2 Clinical Research Center, National Hospital Organization Nagasaki Medical Center, Ohmura, Nagasaki, Japan

*Address all correspondence to: inazumahayato7@gmail.com

References

[1] Whitehead A, Cataldo PA. Technical considerations in stoma creation. Clinics in Colon and Rectal Surgery. 2017;**30**(3):162-171

[2] Watson MJ, Kundu N, Coppa C, Djohan R, Hashimoto K, Eghtesad B, et al. Role of tissue expanders in patients with loss of abdominal domain awaiting intestinal transplantation. Transplant International. 2013;**26**(12):1184-1190

[3] Delaney CP, Fazio VW. Ileostomy construction in complex reoperative surgery with associated abdominal wall defects. American Journal of Surgery. 2000;**180**(1):51-52

[4] Yezhelyev MV, Deigni O, Losken A. Management of full-thickness abdominal wall defects following tumor resection. Annals of Plastic Surgery. 2012;**69**(2):186-191

[5] Stone HH, Fabian TC, Turkleson ML, Jurkiewicz MJ. Management of acute full-thickness losses of abdominal wall. Annals of Surgery. 1981;**193**:612-618

[6] Cederna JP, Davies BW. Total abdominal wall reconstruction. Annals of Plastic Surgery. 1990;**25**:65-70

[7] Fujioka M, Miyazato O, Yamamoto T, Nishimura G. Full thickness rectus abdominis muscle defect due to the contact burn. Burns. 2002;**28**:391-393

[8] Kendrick JH, Casali RE, Lang NP, Read RC. The complicated septic abdominal wound. Archives of Surgery. 1982;**117**(4):464-468

[9] Ali F, Safawi EB, Zakaria Z, Basiron N. Abdominal wall reconstruction after resection of an enterocutaneous fistula with an island pedicled anterolateral thigh perforator flap. Case report. La Clinica Terapeutica. 2013;**164**(5):413-415

[10] Slade DA, Carlson GL. Takedown of enter cutaneous fistula and complex abdominal wall reconstruction. The Surgical Clinics of North America. 2013;**93**(5):1163-1183

[11] Meguid MM, McIvor A, Xenos L. Creation of a neoabdominal wall to facilitate emergency placement of a terminal ileostomy in a morbidly obese patient. American Journal of Surgery. 1997;**173**(4):298-300

[12] Steinhagen E, Colwell J, Lisa M. Intestinal stomas—Postoperative stoma care and peristomal skin complications. Clinics in Colon and Rectal Surgery. 2017;**30**(3):184-192

[13] Carlsen BT, Farmer DG, Busuttil RW, Miller TA, Rudkin GH. Incidence and management of abdominal wall defects after intestinal and multivisceral transplantation. Plastic and Reconstructive Surgery. 2007;**119**:1247-1255

[14] Fazio VW. Crohn's disease. In: Keighley MRB, Pemberton JH, Fazio VW, Parc R, editors. Atlas of Colorectal Surgery. New York: Churchill Livingston; 1996. pp. 61-91

[15] Atema JJ, Furnée EJ, Maeda Y, Warusavitarne J, Tanis PJ, Bemelman WA, et al. Major complex abdominal wall repair in contaminated fields with use of a non-cross-linked biologic mesh: A dual-institutional experience. World Journal of Surgery. 2017;**41**(8):1993-1999

[16] Connolly PT, Teubner A, Lees NP, Anderson ID, Scott NA, Carlson GL. Outcome of reconstructive surgery for intestinal fistula in the open abdomen. Annals of Surgery. 2008;**247**(3):440-444

[17] Asham E, Uknis C, Rastellini C, Elias G, Cicalese L. Acellular dermal

matrix provides a good option for abdominal wall closure following small bowel transplantation: A case report. Transplantation Proceedings. 2006;**38**:1770-1771

[18] Zanfi C, Cescon M, Lauro A, et al. Incidence and management of abdominal closure-related complications in adult intestinal transplantation. Transplantation. 2008;**85**:1607-1609

[19] Gondolesi G, Selvaggi G, Tzakis A, et al. Use of the abdominal rectus fascia as a nonvascularized allograft for abdominal wall closure after liver, intestinal, and multivisceral transplantation. Transplantation. 2009;**87**:1884-1888

[20] Clifton MS, Heiss KF, Keating JJ, Mackay G, Ricketts RR. Use of tissue expanders in the repair of complex abdominal wall defects. Journal of Pediatric Surgery. 2011;**46**:372-377

[21] de Vries Reilingh TS, van Goor H, Rosman C, Bemelmans MH, de Jong D, van Nieuwenhoven EJ, et al. "Components separation technique" for the repair of large abdominal wall hernias. Journal of the American College of Surgeons. 2003;**196**(1):32

[22] Ramirez OM, Ruas E, Dellon AL. "Components separation" method for closure of abdominal-wall defects: An anatomic and clinical study. Plastic and Reconstructive Surgery. 1990;**86**:519-526

[23] Christy MR, Apostolides J, Rodriguez ED, Manson PN, Gens D, Scalea T. Eplasty. 2012;**12**:e17

[24] Ferreira P, Malheiro E, Choupina M, et al. Gunshot abdominal wall injury reconstructed with an innervated latissimus dorsi free flap. The Journal of Trauma. 2007;**63**:691-695

[25] Wong CH, Lin CH, Fu B, Fang JF. Reconstruction of complex abdominal wall defects with free flaps: Indications and clinical outcome. Plastic and Reconstructive Surgery. 2009;**124**:500-509

[26] Kayano S, Sakuraba M, Miyamoto S, Nagamatsu S, Taji M, Umezawa H, et al. Comparison of pedicled and free anterolateral thigh flaps for reconstruction of complex defects of the abdominal wall: Review of 20 consecutive cases. Journal of Plastic, Reconstructive & Aesthetic Surgery. 2012;**65**(11):1525-1529

[27] Williams JK, Carlson GW, dsChalain T, Howel R, Coleman JJ. Role of tensor fasciae latae in abdominal wall reconstruction. Plastic and Reconstructive Surgery. 1998;**101**:713-718

[28] Koshima I, Fujitsu M, Ushio S, Sugiyama N, Yamashita S. Flow-through anterior thigh flaps with a short pedicle for reconstruction of lower leg and foot defects. Plastic and Reconstructive Surgery. 2005;**115**(1):155-162

[29] Ao M, Nagase Y, Mae O, Namba Y. Reconstruction of posttraumatic defects of the foot by flow-through anterolateral or anteromedial thigh flaps with preservation of posterior tibial vessels. Annals of Plastic Surgery. 1997;**38**:598-603

[30] Fujioka M, Hayashida K, Morooka S, Saijou H, Nonaka T. Combined serratus anterior and latissimus dorsi myocutaneous flap for obliteration of an irradiated pelvic exenteration defect and simultaneous site for colostomy revision. World Journal of Surgical Oncology. 2014;**12**(1):319-323

[31] Strawberry CW, Jacobs JS, McCraw JB. Reconstruction for cervical irradiation ulcers with my cutaneous flaps. Head & Neck Surgery. 1984;**6**(4):836-841

[32] Calderon W, Chang N, Mathes SJ. Comparison of the effect of bacterial

inoculation in musculocutaneous and fasciocutaneous flaps. Plastic and Reconstructive Surgery. 1986;77:785-792

[33] Russell RC, Graham DR, Feller AM, et al. Experimental evaluation of the antibiotic carrying capacity of a muscle flap into a fibrotic cavity. Plastic and Reconstructive Surgery. 1988;**81**:162-168

[34] Rudolph R, Arganese T, Woodward M. The ultrastructure and etiology of chronic radiotherapy damage in human skin. Annals of Plastic Surgery. 1982;**9**(4):282-292

[35] Schaverien M, Saint-Cyr M. Perforators of the lower leg: Analysis of perforator locations and clinical application for pedicled perforator flaps. Plastic and Reconstructive Surgery. 2008;**122**:161-170

[36] Taylor GI, Pan WR. Angiosomes of the leg: Anatomic study and clinical implications. Plastic and Reconstructive Surgery. 1998;**102**:599-616

[37] Carriquiry C, Aparecida Costa M, Vasconez LO. An anatomic study of the septocutaneous vessels of the leg. Plastic and Reconstructive Surgery. 1985;**76**:354-363

[38] Parrett BM, Matros E, Pribaz JJ, et al. Lower extremity trauma: Trends in the management of soft-tissue reconstruction of open tibia-fibula fractures. Plastic and Reconstructive Surgery. 2006;**117**:1315-1322

[39] El-Sabbagh AH. Skin perforator flaps: An algorithm for leg reconstruction. Journal of Reconstructive Microsurgery. 2011;**27**:511-523

[40] Sameem M, Au M, Wood T, Farrokhyar F, Mahoney J. A systematic review of complication and recurrence rates of musculocutaneous, fasciocutaneous, and perforator-based flaps for treatment of pressure sores. Plastic and Reconstructive Surgery. 2012;**130**(1):67e-77e

[41] Ragoowansi R, Yii N, Niranjan N. Immediate vulvar and vaginal reconstruction using the gluteal-fold flap: Long-term results. British Journal of Plastic Surgery. 2004;**57**(5):406-410

[42] Fujioka M, Hayashida K, Murakami C. Resurfacing patella using pedicled soleus perforator flap. Techniques in Knee Surgery. 2012;**11**(3):147-150

Chapter 3

Intestinal Ostomy Complications and Care

Francielle Profeta Rodrigues, Jane Andrea Vieira Novaes, Marcela Monteiro Pinheiro, Paula Martins and José Renan Cunha-Melo

Abstract

The management of patients submitted to intestinal stomas (ileostomy or colostomy) and description of the routine care and main complications are the scope of the chapter. The impact of the stoma on patients' daily life with a functional list of capabilities they can exert with security and illustrations of the commonest drawbacks are also discussed. A series of pictures showing the most commonly occurring complications depicted in the section Problems and complications help to a better understanding of the author's intended message. Finally in the "References" topic, it was tried to cite society-based guidelines and review papers concerning ostomy care and complications.

Keywords: colostomy and ileostomy management, complications, peristomal hernia, prolapse, retraction, necrosis

1. Introduction

An ostomy is a surgically created opening between a hollow organ and the body surface or between two hollow organs. The surgical interventions which result in ostomies are based on the need to modify the natural way of ingestion of food or excretion of waste products. The word *ostomy* comes from the Latin word *ostium*, meaning mouth or opening, plus the suffix *-tomy*, implying a surgical or injury state. The word *stoma* comes from the Greek word for mouth and is used interchangeably with ostomy.

Depending on the organ involved, an ostomy is further characterized by adding the name of the organ involved: gastrostomy to indicate an opening from the stomach to the skin, an ileostomy from the ileum to the skin, and a colostomy from the colon. In addition an anastomosis between the small bowel and colon is called *ileocolostomy*; between sigmoid colon and the rectum, a *sigmoidorectostomy*; and between the stomach and the jejunum, a *gastrojejunostomy*. A loop ostomy is built by bringing a loop of bowel through the skin and then dividing the antimesenteric border and maturing it so that there are two open lumens, the proximal and the distal.

An ostomy can be created virtually anywhere along the gastrointestinal tract. For diversion of the fecal stream, the most common ostomies involve the distal small intestine (ileostomy) and large intestine (colostomy).

Temporary or permanent fecal diversions by the creation of an ostomy, which is a purposeful anastomosis between a segment of the gastrointestinal tract and the skin of the anterior abdominal wall, may be needed to manage a variety of

 IntechOpen

pathologic conditions, including congenital anomalies, colon obstruction, inflammatory bowel disease, traumatic disruption of the intestinal tract, or gastrointestinal malignancy, when restoration of intestinal continuity is contraindicated or not immediately feasible given the patient's clinical condition. End ostomy is the name indicative of a hollow viscera pull to the skin as a terminal opening. In this way only one open lumen is viewed. The majority of ostomies today are created as a temporary measure, although the ostomies with a permanent intention are not rare. Construction of an ostomy should always be performed using a segment of healthy, well-vascularized bowel. Expected difficulties arise in morbidly obese patients or those with extensive adhesions.

This chapter will discuss ostomies brought to the surface of the body, focusing primarily on ileostomy and colostomy complications with the proposed treatment approach.

Even when the stoma is technically adequate, alterations on the corporal image, lifestyle, and sexuality, as well as the need for auto care may occur leading to social and psychological disturbances which difficult the individual social adaptation [1].

2. Ostomy planning

2.1 Counseling

The multiple aspects involved in rehabilitation of patients with an ostomy including the medical and nursing care must be initiated at the moment of the indication and extended until a complete adaptation of the patient with the new situation occurs.

Preoperative preparation prior to planned ostomy creation includes stoma site selection, emotional support, and patient education, as well as early planning for subsequent discharge, ongoing rehabilitation care for the patient and family, and outpatient follow-up.

Patients who require an ostomy for fecal diversion often experience physical, psychological, and emotional stress related to misconceptions and fears regarding social acceptance, sexuality, and economic burden. To allay these fears, preoperative education, counseling, and ostomy site selection should be undertaken, whenever possible, from a skilled ostomy nurse specialist. Several aspects going from the initial patient's approach with clarification of doubts about diagnosis, familiar history, intestinal habit, medicines, social activities, emotional state, psychomotor skills, and schooling to skin conditions' evaluation are important to provide a proper knowledge about the medical condition and adequately educate the patient. To achieve the autonomy about the ostomy care, the patient should be oriented toward maintaining a well-recognized standard of care, with decrease of complications. In addition to improved overall quality of life, preoperative counseling is associated with decreased stoma-related postoperative complications, improved postoperative patient stoma proficiency, and earlier discharge from the hospital [2, 3].

2.2 Site selection and marking

Proper site selection is essential for minimizing postoperative complications and achieving a good postoperative quality of life. A poor site selection is more likely in patients undergoing emergency surgery compared with elective surgery. Obesity, scars, type of surgery (emergency or elective), underlying disease,

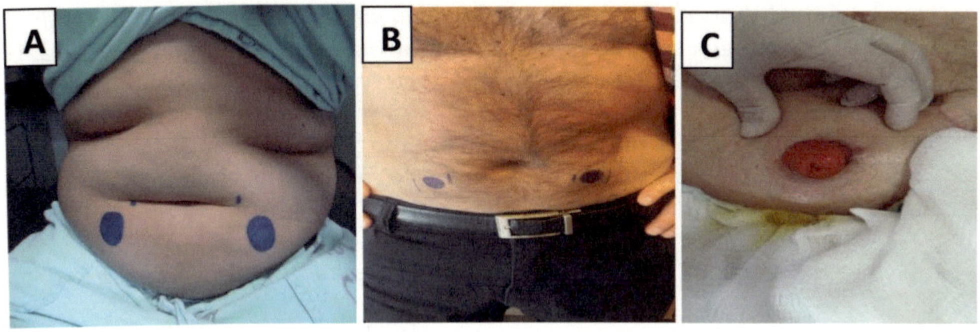

Figure 1.
Stoma site demarcation. This is an important step to achieve a technically good result after ostomy confection allowing adequate pouch adaptation, especially in obese patients with skin folds (A), permitting the natural wear of belts and cloths (B). The ideal appearance of an ostomy is depicted at C.

abdominal wall contour (sitting and standing), prior abdominal incisions, bony prominences, occupation, clothing style, and physical activity impairment can be cited as factors which difficult the adequate site of an abdominal stoma [4] (**Figure 1A** and **B**).

Once selected the ostomy site, laparoscopic approach is a safe and effective alternative to laparotomy for creating a loop ostomy. The advantages of the laparoscopic approach are that it provides an excellent view of the abdominal cavity and minimizes the risks and complications of an open procedure. Whatever surgical approach is used, the goal is to obtain a stoma technically in good conditions in order to prevent complications (**Figure 1C**).

3. Intestinal ostomies: routine care

Many pouching systems are available, as either one- or two-piece systems. The main functions of ostomy pouches are to contain the ostomy effluent, contain odor, and protect the peristomal skin. The patient should be taught strategies that can help promote pouch adherence to the skin and minimize leakage. Occasional leakage is common and is nothing to be concerned about. However, if the leak is constant, a double check of the stoma bag is advisable. A stoma leakage usually results from a stoma bag that has not been fitted correctly leaving gaps in the wafer and the hole does not fit snugly around the stoma. If this happens an ostomate nurse should be contacted for advice and eventual adjustments [5].

3.1 Protecting the peristomal skin

The protection of peristomal skin is better achieved with simple measures such as:

1. Selecting a bag system that conforms to the abdominal contour at the stoma location

2. Sizing the opening of the barrier ring to minimize the amount of exposed skin

3. Using adjunctive products to improve the fixation of the pouch (adhesive agents, Skin Prep) and to prevent irritation and injury of the skin (skin barrier paste and powder)

The abdominal skin around the stoma should always look the same as the skin anywhere else on the abdomen. Ostomy output can make this skin tender or sore. To prevent skin dermatitis, the American Cancer Society recommends:

1. Use the right size pouch and skin barrier opening. An opening that's too small can cut or injure the stoma and may cause it to swell. If the opening is too large, output could get to and irritate the skin.

2. Change the pouching system regularly to avoid leaks and skin irritation.

3. Do not rip the pouching system away from the skin or remove it more than once a day unless there's a problem.

4. Clean the skin around the stoma with water, and dry the skin completely before putting on a skin barrier or adapting the pouch.

5. Watch for sensitivities and allergies (to the adhesive, skin barrier, paste, tape, or pouch material).

6. Patch testing different products for skin sensitivity or allergies.

Loop ileostomies are typically more difficult to manage than end ileostomies because the stoma frequently empties close to the skin surface [6].

3.2 Emptying and changing the ostomy pouching system

It is important that the patient be taught how to change and empty the pouching system before leaving the hospital. The use of sterile supplies is not necessary. Toilet paper, facial tissue, or paper towels can be used to clean around the stoma instead of sterile gauze pads.

3.3 How to empty the pouch

Odor and gas are common concerns for any individual with an ostomy.

The patient should be assured that ostomy pouches are odor-proof, but when the pouch is emptied, odor is normal. Simple strategies can help reduce odor.

I. To keep bulging and leaking, it's recommended emptying the ostomy pouch when it is about 1/3 full. To empty the pouch, the patient should adopt the following steps:

   1. Sit as far back on the toilet as you can or on a chair facing the toilet.

   2. Place a small strip of toilet paper in the toilet to decrease splashing.

   3. Hold the bottom of the pouch up and open the clip at the end or tail of the pouch.

   4. Slowly unroll the tail over the toilet.

   5. Gently empty the contents.

   6. Clean the outside and inside of the pouch tail with toilet paper.

7. Roll up the end of the pouch and clip.

8. Change the pouch one to two times weekly and as needed for any signs of leakage, itching, or burning of the peristomal skin.

9. Keep the tail of the pouch clean so that it does not become a source of odor. This can be accomplished by everting the tail of a pouch prior to emptying it.

10. Use a room spray or pouch deodorant to minimize odor associated with emptying.

3.4 Time to change the pouching system

Different pouching systems are made to last different lengths of time. Some are changed every day, some every 3 days or so, and some just once a week. It depends on the type of pouch used. There may be less bowel activity at certain times of the day. It's easiest to change the pouching system during these times. Every patient establishes its own preference about the proper time to change the pouch. Some prefer early morning before breakfast and some allow at least 1 h after a meal. Right after surgery, ostomy output may be thin and watery and the bowel discharges unpredictable. As the output gets thicker, it becomes easier to select the best time for changing.

3.5 The pouching system seal

The pouching system must stick to the skin. It's important to change it before it loosens or leaks. The length of time a pouch will stay sealed to the skin depends on many things, such as the weather, skin condition, scars, weight changes, diet, activity, body shape near the stoma, and the nature of the ostomy output.

Other factors may affect how long a pouch sticks to the skin. Among them it can be cited:

1. Sweating will shorten the number of days the pouching system can be worn.

2. Body heat and outside temperature cause skin barriers to loosen more quickly than usual.

3. Moist, oily skin may reduce wearing time.

4. Weight changes will affect how long you can wear a pouch. Gaining or losing weight after stoma surgery can change the abdominal shape with need for use of an entirely different system.

5. Diet may affect the seal. Foods that cause watery output are more likely to break a seal than a thicker discharge.

6. Physical activities may affect wearing time. Swimming, very strenuous sports, or anything that intensifies sweat may shorten wear time [7].

3.6 Bathing

To take a shower is possible with or without a pouching system in place. Normal exposure to air or contact with soap and water will not harm the stoma. Water will not flow into the stoma. Soap will not irritate it, but soap may interfere with the skin barrier sticking to the skin. Taking a bath without the pouching system is however highly impractical for the most obvious of reasons, primarily the risk of fecal output while bathing, which cannot be controlled. It's best to only use water while cleaning the skin around your stoma. If soap is used, one must be sure to rinse the skin well.

3.7 Shaving hair under the pouch

Having a lot of hair around the stoma can make it hard to get the skin barrier to stick well and may cause pain when the pouch is removed. It is advisable whenever possible to trim instead of shaving with a blade the skin hairs around the stoma to prevent skin scarification and inflammatory reaction. However if the hair density is high and shaving is indicated, it is recommended a dry shave of the skin around the stoma with stoma powder, since soap and shaving creams have lotions and oils that may impair the skin barrier sticking. After shaving, the skin must be rinsed well and dried before applying a pouch.

3.8 What to wear when having a colostomy

No special clothes for everyday wear are needed. Ostomy pouches are fairly flat and hard to see under most clothing. The pressure of elastic undergarments will not harm the stoma or prevent bowel function.

If the ostomate gains weight after the ostomy surgery, this can affect the clothes he was used to more than the pouching system itself.

Snug undergarments such as cotton stretch underpants, T-shirts, or camisoles may give an extra support, security, and help conceal pouches. A simple pouch cover adds comfort by absorbing body sweat and keeps the plastic pouch from resting against your skin. Men can wear either boxer or jockey-type shorts.

4. Ostomy problems and complications

The construction of an intestinal stoma should not be considered a trivial undertaking. Serious complications requiring immediate reoperations can occur, as can minor problems that will subject the patient to daily and nightly distress. Intestinal stomas undoubtedly will dramatically change lifestyles. Patients will experience physiologic and psychologic detriment with stoma-related problems [8].

- Activities

A common concern for many patients is the impact of the stoma on activities of daily living. The patient can be reassured that most activities can be safely resumed with minimal, if any, modifications. As an example, bathing and showering can be performed with the pouch on or off, and clothing modifications are generally not required. Most sports activities can be resumed as well, with the exception of extreme contact sports, which could potentially damage the stoma. The addition of a belt or binder is helpful in maintaining a pouch seal during vigorous activity and with perspiration.

- Sex

Sexual activity is a particular concern for many patients with an ostomy. Patient counseling should address questions regarding sexual activity and partner response. The ostomy by itself does not affect organic sexual function; however it is advised to empty the pouch and assure an intact pouch seal before engaging in sexual activity [9].

- Travel

Patients who are traveling should be advised to take extra ostomy supplies, to avoid exposing ostomy pouches and adhesives to extreme temperatures, which may alter the adhesive quality, and drink only bottled water if tap water is not known to be safe.

4.1 Risk factors for stomal complications

The main risk factors for the occurrence of stoma complications are:

1. Age.

2. Comorbidity—inflammatory bowel diseases, diverticulitis.

3. Obesity.

4. Precocious physical effort.

5. Stoma type—ileostomies are more prone for the complication occurrence than colostomy or gastrostomy.

6. Stoma protrusion.

7. Type of surgery—emergency surgery is more likely to evolute with complication.

8. Stoma site—lack of preoperative demarcation leading to inadequate stoma placement.

9. Quality of stomal bag devices.

10. Inadequate stoma care—the ideal care is provided by specialized nurse.

4.2 Functional complications

- Output

Patients with colostomy or ileostomy experiment physiologic changes related to the loss of continence and reduced ileal and colonic absorptive surface area with consequent fluid and electrolyte balance disturbances and lifestyle adaptation but generally with little effect on nutrition. It should be emphasized that if more than 50 cm terminal ileum is resected, nutritional consequences are likely to occur [10].

Ostomy output is related to the location of the opening in the bowel, as the more proximal the ostomy, the less surface area is available for water and electrolyte absorption and so the more liquid the stools. Right-sided colostomies, for example, not only produce a high volume but also have the additional disadvantage of a malodorous output because of the effects of colonic bacteria.

The type and volume of output (effluent), and therefore fluid loss, are determined by the location of the stoma relative to the ileocecal valve. Ileostomies, cecostomies, and ascending colostomies typically produce output (effluent) >500 mL/day that contains digestive enzymes, which is irritating to the mucosa and skin, while descending/sigmoid colostomies produce stool that does not contain digestive enzymes.

The output from an ileostomy tends to be fairly watery and green or bilious in color. Within a few weeks of resumption of a regular diet, the material becomes thicker and more yellow-brown, with a watery porridge or applesauce consistency. Depending on the amount of small bowel removed, the output is looser, and the patient is more prone to dehydration. Most ileostomates notice little odor from the output, but, certain foods (e.g., eggs and fish) may produce an offensive smell.

The ostomy output is also affected by diet, fluid intake, medications, and organic problems such as Crohn's disease or adhesions. Diarrhea, frequent loose or watery bowel movements in greater amounts, than expected, is a warning that something is not right. It can come suddenly and may cause cramps. The causes of diarrhea are variable: diet, emotional stress, intestinal infection, antibiotics, and short bowel syndrome.

- Volume

In a healthy individual, 1000–2000 mL of fluid passes through the ileocecal valve daily. This volume is reduced to 100–200 mL in normal stool as it passes through the colon. So a left-sided colostomy output is similar in volume and composition to the feces that would be passed transanally. The volume of ileostomy output varies fairly widely among patients but only mildly from day to day in a single individual. In the early postoperative period, the ileostomy output is 1000–1500 ml/day. In a few days, this volume is reduced to about 500 ml, even with no dietary restrictions; however it is known that fatty food and large amounts of liquid increase transit and the fluidity of the effluent.

- Transit

Resection of anus and/or colon affects the function of the proximal GI tract and the integration of endocrine and neuroenteric activities. It seems that small bowel transit time decrease after ileostomy due to adaptation to the new condition whose mechanisms are not yet well understood.

Microbial flora of an individual is fairly stable over time, whereas there is great variability among individuals. After creation of an ileostomy, the distal ileum is rapidly colonized with a variety of bacteria.

- Nutrition

The colon has little role in the maintenance of normal nutrition, working primarily to absorb fluid and to store feces. Thus, removal of the colon has little effect on nutrition. However, loss of part of the terminal ileum may result in loss of bile acids and poor absorption of fat and fat-soluble vitamins. Vitamin B12 may also not be adequately absorbed in patients with terminal ileal loss that may result in pernicious or macrocytic anemia requiring monthly administration of vitamin B12. Absorption may also be impeded by ileal bacterial overgrowth. Kidney stones may be a consequence of chronic dehydration and acid urine. Adding sodium bicarbonate to the diet and increasing fluid intake may help to prevent uric acid stone formation.

4.3 Technical and anatomic stoma-related complications

Proper creation, management, and closure of ostomy are critical both for the treatment of specific disorders and for the peace of mind of the patient. A poor site selection contributes to the rate of stomal complications and is more likely to occur in patients undergoing emergency surgery compared with elective surgery. Other risk factors for stomal problems include:

- Height of stoma <10 mm
- Tobacco usage
- Comorbid conditions (obesity, inflammatory bowel disease, diabetes)

The rates for stomal complications range from 14 to 79%. Peristomal dermatitis is the most common complication. Other complications include poor stoma siting, high output, ischemia, retraction, parastomal hernia formation, stomal stenosis, bleeding, and prolapse. Surgeons should be cognizant of these complications before, during, and after stoma creation, and adequate measures should be taken to avoid them [11].

Stomal and peristomal complications can occur in the early postoperative period or many years later. Complications occurring in the course of days after surgery are often related to technical issues. Those occurring within 3 months of stoma construction—necrosis, bleeding, retraction, and mucocutaneous separation—are more frequently related to suboptimal stoma site selection. Late stomal complications are generally described for permanent ostomies and include parastomal hernia, stomal prolapse, and stenosis. The site of closure of the ostomy can be associated with complications such as delayed healing, infection, and hernia formation.

Loop ileostomies have higher complication rates when compared to end colostomy or end ileostomy and with loop colostomy. The most common problems of end and loop ileostomies are dehydration, skin irritation, and small bowel obstruction. Prolapse can occur in all types of stomas but is more prevalent in loop colostomies, especially those constructed using the transverse colon.

4.4 Time-related complications

I. Immediate—occurring up to 24 h after stoma placement. The more common immediate complications are edema, bleeding, ischemia, and necrosis.

II. Early—occur 1–15 days after surgery. The more common are retraction, mucocutaneous detachment, peristomal evisceration, and peristomal fistula.

III. Late—occur from 15 days to months after surgery. Retraction, stenosis, prolapse, granuloma, and peristomal hernia are examples of the more important late complications.

4.4.1 Peristomal skin complications

I. Dermatitis

II. Venous varices

III. Pseudoverrucous lesions

IV. Bacterial and fungal infections

4.4.2 When the ostomate should call the doctor or ostomy nurse

- Cramps lasting more than 2 or 3 h
- Continuous nausea and vomiting
- No ostomy output for 4–6 h with cramping and nausea
- Severe watery discharge lasting more than 5 or 6 h
- Bad odor lasting more than a week (this may be a sign of infection.)
- A cut in the stoma
- Injury to the stoma
- Bad skin irritation or deep sores (ulcers)
- A lot of bleeding from the stoma opening (or a moderate amount in the pouch that you notice several times when emptying it)
- Continuous bleeding where the stoma meets the skin
- Unusual change in your stoma size or color
- Anything unusual going on with your ostomy

The complication occurrence in intestinal stomas might be related to factors such as lack of demarcation of the skin site, surgical technique itself, or to postoperative care. Each type of complication deserves a different treatment approach. For sure a prompt intervention is advisable to avoid or to minimize the complication occurrence.

5. Illustration of more common ostomy complications

The more common type of ostomy complications are:

1. Mucosal edema
2. Peristomal dermatitis
3. Retraction
4. Ostomy prolapse
5. Mucosal/skin detachment
6. Hematoma

7. Necrosis

8. Parastomal hernia

9. Stenosis

The following pictures are illustrative examples of these complications.

5.1 Mucosal edema

On the practical settings, edema may not be considered as a true complication as it can result from a normal physiological response after manipulation of intestinal loop. It is normal for the stoma to be edematous postoperatively looking swollen within 4–6 hours. The swelling progresses for the first 2 days and by the fifth day subsides markedly. The edema continues to decrease for the first 6–8 weeks after surgery. While edematous, the stomal mucosa is pale and translucent and the stoma tissue remains soft. The main approach to treat an ostomy edema is observation plus the care with manipulation and correct application of pouch, to avoid mechanical trauma. It should be reminded that if the edema is caused by technical problems, e.g., a narrowed abdominal wall opening, it may be advisable to reoperate in order to correct the problem [11] (**Figure 2**).

5.2 Peristomal dermatitis

Peristomal dermatitis is the most common stoma complication. It is characterized by skin irritation around the stoma, caused by several factors: irritation of the skin by feces, contact or products used in ostomy care which may be corrosive, contact allergy due to the nature of the chemical component of the pouch in contact with the skin, mechanical infection by pouch withdrawal-induced trauma or by compression of the fixation belt, and bacterial or fungal skin infection caused by humidity and effluent from gut making the peristomal skin more vulnerable to microorganisms' proliferation. The most common symptoms are itching, burning sensation, and pain. Diabetic, immunocompromised, and long-term use of antibiotics increase the risk of infectious dermatitis in patients with intestinal stomas [12, 13] (**Figure 3**).

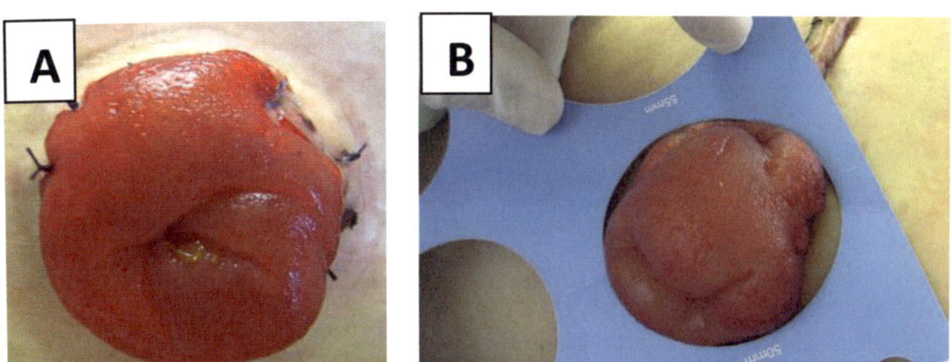

Figure 2.
Ileostomy edema. Usual appearance; (B) care to apply the bag avoiding trauma. The stoma measurement selected for the pouching system should allow for an opening 1/8 inch to prevent stoma necrosis.

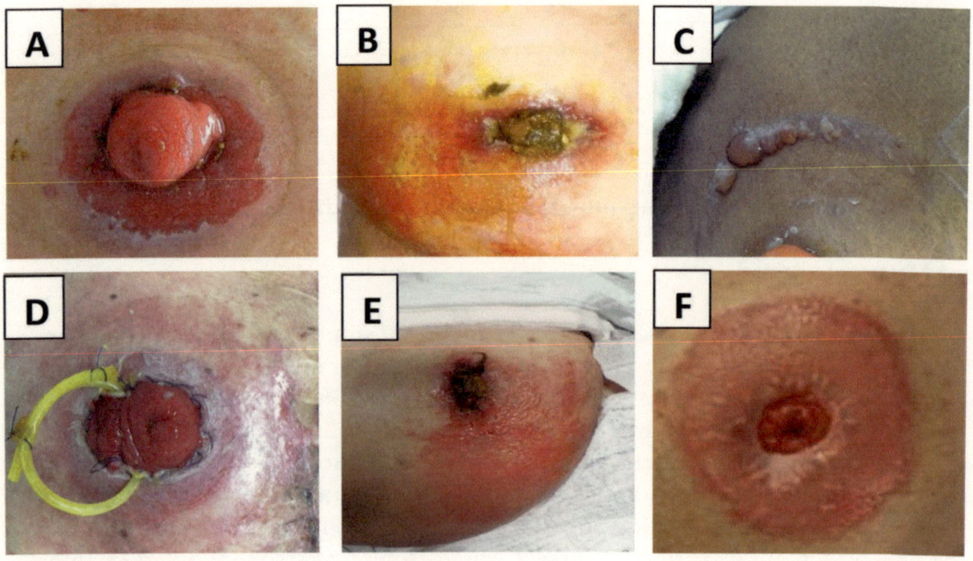

Figure 3.
Peristomal dermatitis. Irritation caused by the effluent in an inadequate pouch adaptation to the skin allowing the prolonged feces/skin contact (A) and an early pouch detachment (B). Blister at the adhesive area in the periphery of pouch resin itself (C). Dermatitis caused by both pouch resin and peripheral adhesive (D). Dermatitis due to contact of feces with skin (E). Fungal dermatitis (F).

5.3 Retraction

A stoma normally protrudes slightly above the skin level being more evident in ileostomies than in colostomies. A retraction of the stoma occurs when the stoma lays flat to the skin or below the skin surface level. Retraction has been reported to occur in as many as 10–24% of all ostomates, can be partial involving the skin and subcutaneous tissue or complete when the stoma is below the level of the fascia, can occur early or late after ostomy, and may result from a poor surgical stoma construction with consequent exteriorization of intestinal loop under tension, insufficient stomal length, poor fixation of the loop to the abdominal wall, or lack of ostomy support. It can also be secondary to abdominal structure anomalies such as thick abdominal wall related to edema, distention, or obesity. The premature removal of the loop device to support the intestine outside the abdominal wall may also contribute to this complication as well as the later scar formation secondary to healing of a mucocutaneous separation or of a necrotic stoma or even chronic peristomal irritation that healed with scar or adhesion at the mucocutaneous junction.

The retraction can become problematic as it can affect the fit of the stoma bag and cause leaks, which can lead to sore and broken skin. This can be rectified by using a stoma bag with a convex wafer to push the stoma forward, an ostomy belt to help support the stoma, and/or barrier rings or a barrier paste to help keep the output off the skin. The depth of retraction may increase with sitting and can vary with peristalsis. Patients with retracted stomas present with effluent undermining the pouching system, persistent leakage, shortened pouch wear time, and resultant peristomal irritant dermatitis [11].

The proper care will depend on a close observation of peristomal area, to prevent worsening of the retraction. The goal of managing a retracted stoma is to maintain a secure seal between the pouch and the skin. Conservative treatment with convex devices attached to the belt and protective skin pastes to fulfill spaces and leveling the interface skin/stoma may solve most cases, but surgical revision should be indicated when a good pouching seal cannot be obtained and skin irritation persists. It should be reminded that complete circumferential mucocutaneous separation accompanied with stomal retraction below the fascia may be a surgical emergency as it can lead to peritonitis (**Figure 4**).

5.4 Prolapse

Prolapse is the term used to describe the telescoping out of the bowel through the stoma. As a consequence the stoma lengthens and becomes more susceptible to abrasion or infection. Prolapse can be partial or complete, and either the distal or the proximal segment of the loop ostomy may prolapse being the distal portion of the bowel the most frequent site to prolapse. The etiology can involve stoma construction difficulties including a weak abdominal wall with poorly developed fascial support; creation of excessively large opening in the abdominal wall; positioning the stoma out of the rectus abdominal muscle; postoperative increase of the abdominal pressure due to obesity, cough, or pregnancy; bowel edema; and inadequate fixation of the bowel to the abdominal wall [14].

Clinically the prolapse increases the size and the length of the stoma and makes the patient's ability to conceal the stoma beneath clothing difficult. Also the edematous stoma bleeds and is more prone to trauma. A prolapsed stoma could also become obstructed making it impossible for feces to pass through what can lead to ischemia and alteration of the color that appears purple or cyanotic. Stomal irritation, bleeding, necrosis, and gangrene of the distal end of the prolapsed stoma may be seen in chronic prolapse. Conservative management includes tender manual reduction of the prolapse, appliance of a hernia type to exert a mild compression, cold dressing to induce vasoconstriction, use of sugar to induce osmotic force to decrease the amount of liquid into the intestinal layers, and ostomate lying down position. The goal of care is to provide a leak-proof pouching system applied while the patient is supine and the prolapse reduced. Surgical correction of prolapse is indicated for definitive ostomies with prediction of long permanence time and involves resection of the prolapse and stoma reconstruction. Temporary prolapse is best treated at the time of reconstruction of intestinal transit [15] (**Figure 5**).

5.5 Mucocutaneous detachment

Mucocutaneous detachment is the separation of the stoma from the peristomal skin. It can be partial with area of separation shallow or deep or circumferential. Usually it is caused by factors such as (a) secondary to retraction or necrosis; (b) sequel of poor healing from an underlying disease process, more commonly in

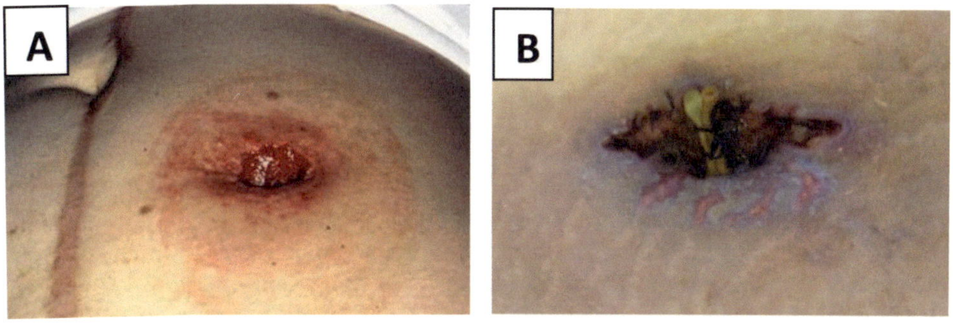

Figure 4.
Ostomy retraction with light (A) and severe inflammatory reaction.

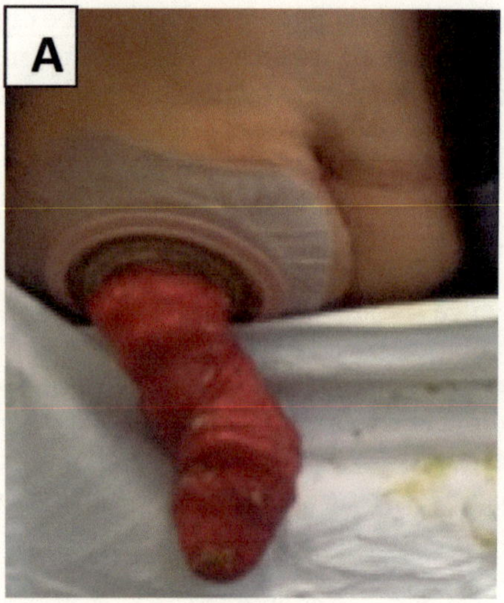

Figure 5.
Stoma prolapse. Note the abnormal length of the stoma. If left untreated the ostomate is more susceptible to abrasions or infection.

the immunocompromised patient related to malnutrition, corticosteroid therapy, diabetes, infection, or post-radiation therapy that result in superficial infection and poor healing; and/or (c) iatrogenic, e.g., creating an oversized opening in the skin when forming the stoma or excessive tension on the suture line, causing a separation of the mucocutaneous junction in the immediate postoperative phase of healing. The ostomate may complain of pain or burning. Assessing the tissue type at the base of the separation often reveals fibrin slough that produces mild to moderate amount of drainage. Stool or urine draining from this site may indicate a fistula. The treatment is conservative consisting of cleaning the wound and use of calcium alginate and hydrofiber. Antibiotics may be indicated for superficial detachment until completion of the healing process. In cases of mucocutaneous separation extending to below the fascia, surgery may be necessary to avoid contamination of the abdominal cavity and peritonitis [11] (**Figure 6**).

5.6 Bleeding and hematoma

The abundant vascularization of the stoma with delicate blood vessels near to the top facilitates bleeding easily. Spots of blood are not a cause for alarm. Cleaning around the stoma as you change the pouch or skin barrier may cause slight bleeding. If the bag has rubbed around the stoma or the blood comes around the edges while the stoma is being cleaned might not be a cause for concern. However if the bleeding is coming from inside the stoma, then it is important to contact your stoma nurse or your doctor for evaluation. The bleeding originating at the mucosal surface will usually stop quickly.

Light bleeding that does not stop spontaneously or excessive bleeding from the stoma usually at the mucocutaneous junction is more frequent in the immediate postoperative period, although it can also occur later. Bleeding may occur due to inadequate hemostasis during stoma construction, portal hypertension, trauma, underlying disease, and because of some medications, such as prolonged use of analgesic anti-inflammatory drugs, blood thinners, and chemotherapy. A correct diagnosis is mandatory to differentiate the mucosal mild trauma-associated bleeding during a pouching system change from other causes that may need even a surgical approach. The adequate treatment will depend on the etiology of bleeding.

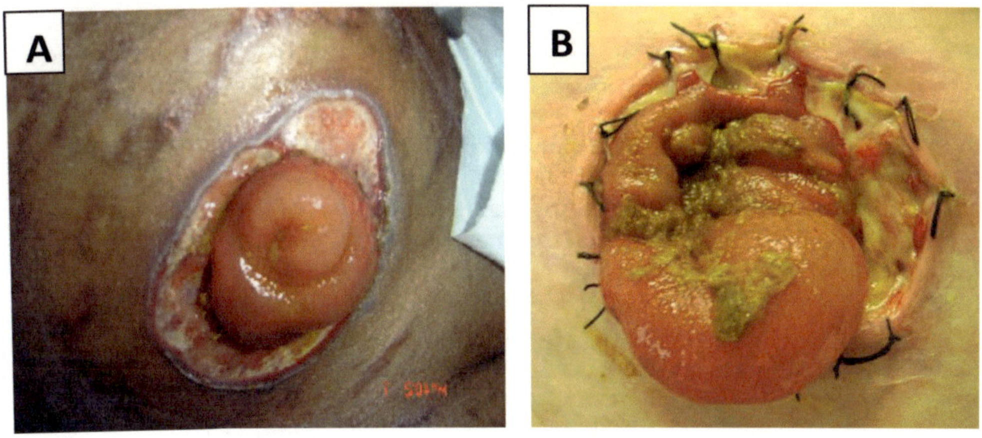

Figure 6.
Mucocutaneous detachment. (A) Usual appearance and (B) mucocutaneous separation due to peristomal infection.

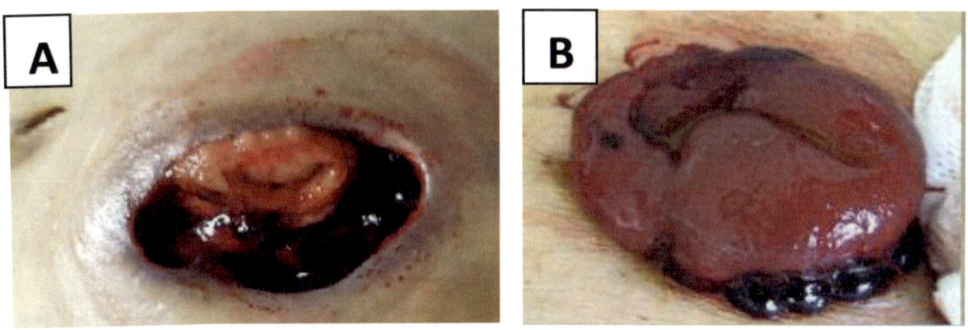

Figure 7.
Bleeding in a mucocutaneous detachment (A) and hematoma at the stoma fixing suture (B).

If the bleeding persists and is superficial and does not stop spontaneously, cauterization, suture placement, topical hemostatic agents (silver nitrate), or direct pressure are required procedures. Frank bleeding presenting as blood that runs down the abdominal wall requires immediate notification of the surgeon. The surgeon removes sutures, lifts the mucosa, secures the vessel with fine forceps, and ligates the bleeder. Portal hypertension induces varices around the stoma resulting in bleeding from the mucocutaneous junction. If severe, it may require sclerotherapy or portosystemic shunting. The most common cause of pharmacological bleeding is the adverse effect of prolonged use of analgesic anti-inflammatory drugs. When bleeding occurs in the late PO period, it may be associated with incorrect use of the ostomy pouch or trauma that can happen following practice of aggressive sports, for example. The management includes the use of compression with a cold dressing. A transparent plastic pouch should be used to permit a direct observation of the stoma allowing quick detection of bleeding or hematoma [15] (**Figure 7**).

5.7 Necrosis

Necrosis may occur when the blood flow to or from the stoma is impaired or interrupted, resulting in severe tissue ischemia with impairment of stoma viability or tissue death. Initially the mucosa turns pale evolving to a purple, brown, and black color. The consistency becomes soft or hard and dry with loss of the characteristic brightness of a normal mucosa. The causes for stoma necrosis are extensive tension on the mesentery, excessive stripping of the mesentery, sutures too narrowly spaced, or constricting sutures. It also can result from interruption of blood flow secondary to embolization or because of abdominal structure anomalies such as thick abdominal wall secondary to edema, distention, or obesity. A higher rate of necrosis has been reported in obese and acutely ill patients.

Observation in cases of superficial or partial (less than one third of circumference) mucosal necrosis is the best approach. Debridement of the necrotic area can define the extension and deepness of necrosis. If the process compromises the whole intestinal wall or extends beyond the aponeurotic plan, a surgical intervention is indicated through the stoma opening or through the main surgical wound if a laparotomy had been performed. The use of two-piece pouch facilitates the daily observation of the stoma with no need of withdrawal of the skin attached piece. Postoperative nursing assessment and management also help prevent potential impairment of a good blood supply to the stoma [11, 16] (**Figure 8**).

5.8 Parastomal hernia

The parastomal hernia, a protrusion of the bowel or loops of intestine through the fascial opening into the subcutaneous tissue around the stoma, occurs months to years after surgery because of surgical technical error or following gradual enlargement of the fascial defect. The incidence rate for parastomal hernia varies with the type and age of the stoma and with surgical technique. It is caused by lack of preoperative demarcation of stoma site with exteriorization outside the rectus abdominal muscle. The main risk factors are intra-abdominal pressure, advanced age, obesity, chronic cough, and long-term use of corticosteroids. If the cause is associated to slight peristomal weakness, a common finding in patients with colostomy, surgical correction is usually not necessary. However some hernias interfere with the proper use of the pouch, and surgery for hernia correction is mandatory [17].

Parastomal hernia presents as a bulge around the stoma and may be partial or circumferential. In supine position the bulge may reduce in size, whereas sitting or standing position, Valsalva maneuver, or cough tends to protrude the hernia, whereas lying down and stoma manual compression intrude the hernia back to the abdomen. The hernia change in position makes the pouching seal more difficult. CT scan with oral contrast confirms the diagnosis. The patient may complain a feeling of discomfort or fullness, and if the stoma incarcerates, the patient presents with an acute obstructed abdomen. The use of support binders when prolonged episodes of

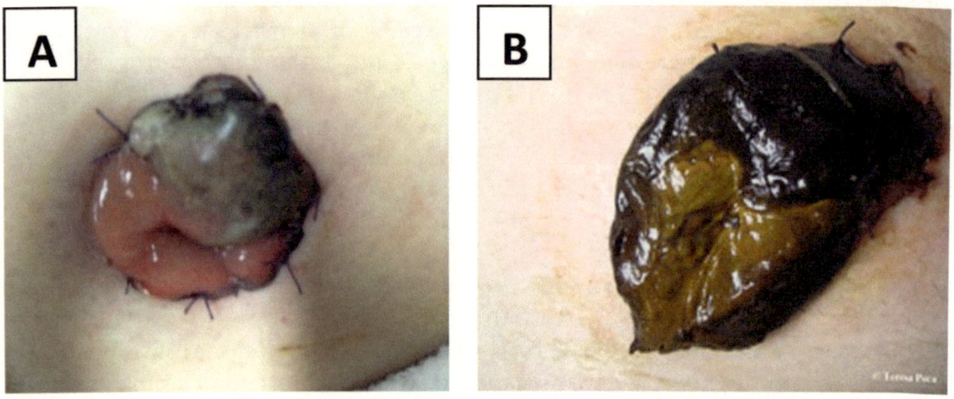

Figure 8.
Stoma necrosis. (A) Partial necrosis; (B) extensive necrosis. An endoscopy is useful to evaluate if the necrosis extends below the level of the fascia. Surgery may be necessary.

increased intra-abdominal pressures are expected (e.g., heavy lifting or hard physical activity) is recommended. Asymptomatic patients can be treated conservatively by the use of support belt or binder, for example, by constipation prevention with diet modification and laxative or stool softener. If signs of obstruction, incarceration, perforation, or recurrent pouching difficulties are present, the patient should be referred to a surgeon. Surgery repair of parastomal hernia can be done by fascial repair, prosthetic mesh, or stoma relocation; however recurrence rates after surgical treatment vary from 33 to 76% [17, 18] (**Figure 9**).

5.9 Stenosis

Stenosis of the stomy opening is characterized by stricture or retraction which makes drainage of the intestinal effluent more difficult. Its incidence is related to the surgical technique itself or as a consequence of precocious complications such as partial necrosis, recurrent inflammatory processes, Crohn's disease, weight gain, and tumor recurrence. The symptoms include abdominal excess of gases, frequent cramps and diarrhea, as well as thin feces. The best option for the treatment of this complication is surgery, but increase of hydric ingestion and eating foods which favor the feces softening may improve the ostomy output [4, 5] (**Figure 10**).

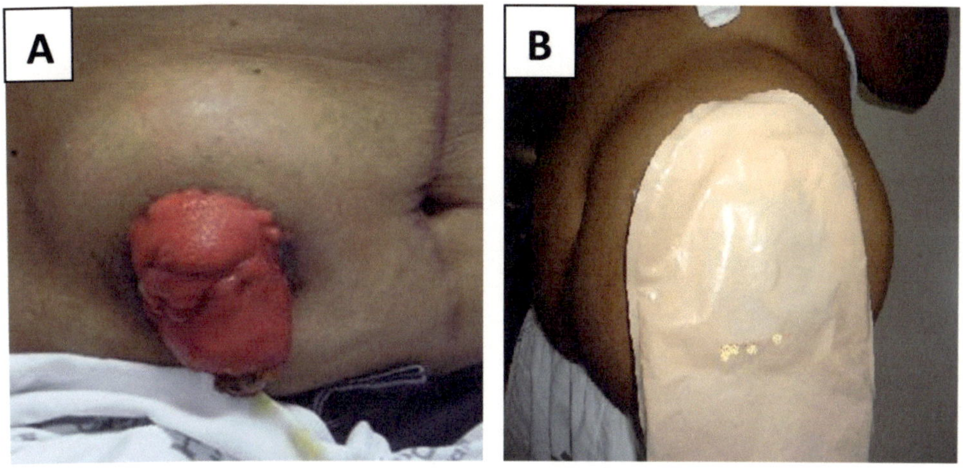

Figure 9.
Parastomal hernia in a prolapsed stoma (A) and a huge parastomal hernia (B).

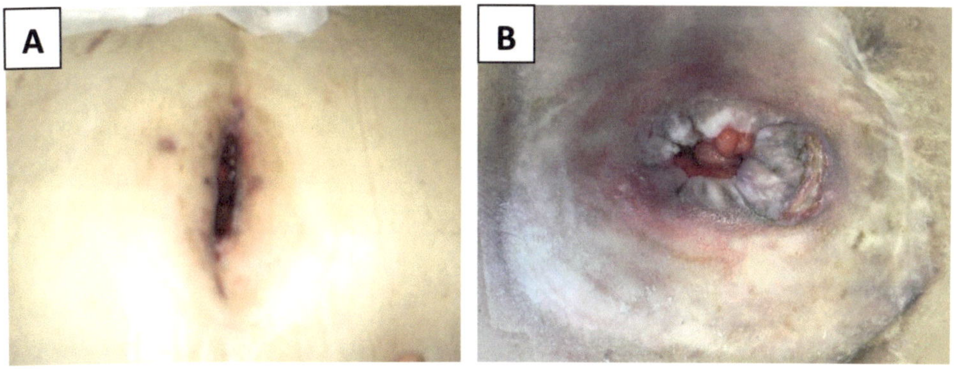

Figure 10.
Stoma stenosis. Note the retraction of skin (A) and the scar tissue around the stoma opening in a chronic stoma stenosis (B).

Author details

Francielle Profeta Rodrigues[1], Jane Andrea Vieira Novaes[1], Marcela Monteiro Pinheiro[1], Paula Martins[2] and José Renan Cunha-Melo[3]*

1 Hospital das Clínicas, Federal University of Minas Gerais (UFMG), Belo Horizonte, MG, Brazil

2 Department of Surgery, School of Medicine, UFMG, Belo Horizonte, MG, Brazil

3 Emeritus of Surgery, Faculty of Medicine, Federal University of Minas Gerais (UFMG), Belo Horizonte, MG, Brasil

*Address all correspondence to: jrcmelo@medicina.ufmg.br

References

[1] Shabbir J, Britton DC. Stoma complications: A literature overview. Colorectal Disease. 2010;**12**:958-964. DOI: 10.1111/j.1463-1318.2009.02006.x

[2] Vonk-Klaassen SM, de Vocht HM, den Ouden MEM, Eddes EH, Schuurmans MJ. Ostomy-related problems and their impact on quality of life of colorectal cancer ostomates: A systematic review. Quality of Life Research. 2016;**25**:125-133. DOI: 10.1007/s11136-015-1050-3

[3] Bass EM, Del Pino A, Tan A, et al. Does preoperative stoma marking and education by the enterostomal therapist affect outcome? Diseases of the Colon and Rectum. 1997;**40**:440-442. DOI: 10.1007/BF02258389

[4] Wound, Ostomy and Continence Nurses Society. WOCN Society and ASCRS Position Statement on Preoperative Stoma Site Marking for Patients Undergoing Colostomy or Ileostomy Surgery. Mt. Laurel, NJ: Author; 2014

[5] Francone TD, Weiser M, Chen W. Overview of Surgical Ostomy for Fecal Diversion. UpToDate, Inc; 2018. https://www.uptodate.com/contents/overview-of-surgical-ostomy-for-fecal-diversion/print?search=colostomy%20 and%20 ileostomy&source=see_link

[6] Wound, Ostomy and Continence Nurses Society. Peristomal Skin Complications: Clinical Resource Guide. Mt. Laurel, NJ: Author. Copyright© 2016 by the Wound, Ostomy and Continence Nurses Society™ (WOCN®); 2016

[7] Burch J. Management of stoma complications. Nursing Times. 2011;**107**(45):17-18. PMID: 22167970

[8] Arumugam PJ, Bevan L, Macdonald L, Watkins AJ, Morgan AR, Beynon J, et al. A prospective audit of stomas-analysis of risk factors and complications and their management. Colorectal Disease. 2003;**5**:49-52. DOI: 10.1046/j.1463-1318.2003.00403.x

[9] Manderson L. Boundary breaches: The body, sex and sexuality after stoma surgery. Social Science and Medicine. 2005;**61**(2):405-415. DOI: 10.1046/j.1463-1318.2003.00403.x

[10] Landmann RG, Weiser M, Chen W. Routine care of patients with an ileostomy or colostomy and management of ostomy complications. www.uptodate.com [last updated February 2017]

[11] Barr JE. Assessment and management of stomal complications: A framework for clinical decision making. Ostomy/Wound Management. 2004;**50**(9):50-67. PMID: 15361633

[12] Meisner S, Lehur P-A, Moran B, Martins L, Jemec GBE. Peristomal skin complications are common, expensive, and difficult to manage: A population based cost modeling study. PLoS ONE. 2012;**7**(5):e37813. DOI: 10.1371/journal.pone.0037813

[13] Nybaek H, Jemec GB. Skin problems in stoma patients. Journal of the European Academy of Dermatology and Venereology. 2010;**24**(3):249-257. DOI: 10.1111/j.1468-3083.2010.03566.x

[14] Kwiatt M, Kawata M. Avoidance and management of stomal complications. Clinics in Colon and Rectal Surgery. 2013;**26**(2):112-121. DOI: 10.1055/s-0033-1348050

[15] Memorial Sloan Kettering Cancer Center. Caring for your ileostomy or colostomy. Available from: https://www.mskcc.org/cancer-care/patient.../caring-for-your-ileostomy-colostomy

[16] Krishnamurty DM, Blatnik J, Mutch M. Stoma complications. Clinics in Colon

and Rectal Surgery. 2017;**30**(3):193-200. DOI: 10.1055/s-0037-1598160

[17] Cima RR, Rosen CW. Parastomal Hernia. UpToDate, Inc.; 2018. https://www.uptodate.com/contents/parastomal-hernia/print?topicRef=15026& source=see_link

[18] Warren JA, Beffa LR, Carbonell AM, et al. Prophylactic placement of permanent synthetic mesh at the time of ostomy closure prevents formation of incisional hernias. Surgery. 2018;**163**:839-846. DOI: 10.1016/j.surg.2017.09.041

Chapter 4

Gastric Microbiota: Between Health and Disease

Hristo Ilianov Iliev, Mila Dimitrova Kovacheva-Slavova, Todor Asenov Angelov, Hristo Yankov Valkov, Ali Bedran and Borislav Georgiev Vladimirov

Abstract

The etiologic link between *H. pylori* infection and gastric chronic inflammation and related complications has been well established, but pathogenic pathways are still widely discussed and not sufficiently clear. The introduction of culture-independent molecular techniques has allowed better understanding of the gastric microbiota and has revealed that, when present, *H. pylori* represents the main colonizer but is part of a far more complex and dynamic microbiota than previously thought. This conceptual shift has made way for new pathogenic theories, focused on the interrelations between *H. pylori* and other gastric microbiota. Main factors that affect the gastric microbiota are gastric acidity, inflammation, and environmental factors, such as diet and drugs. Previous studies have made progress in explaining the complex interactions between gastric microorganisms in healthy individuals and their role in the development of related gastroduodenal (peptic ulcers and gastric cancer (GC)) and extraintestinal diseases, but more scientific proof is needed. This review presents current knowledge on gastric microbiota and its role in health and in the development of gastroduodenal diseases.

Keywords: gastric microbiota, *H. pylori*, pathogenesis, chronic inflammation, peptic ulcers, gastric cancer

1. Introduction

The first isolation of *Helicobacter pylori* (*H. pylori*) in 1982 [1] changed the traditional misconception that the stomach, with its naturally hostile environment, cannot be a reservoir for microbial species. Since then *H. pylori* has been well established as a key factor in gastric pathology, being the main cause of chronic active gastritis. This inflammation can progress to often interlinked severe complications such as atrophic gastritis, peptic ulcer disease, and gastric malignancies [2]. The assumption of the uniqueness of *H. pylori* as the only bacteria able to survive in the gastric hostile environment has also fast been shattered with the advances in culture-dependent and culture-independent techniques that revealed that *H. pylori* is part of a complex gastric microbiota. The gastric microbial density is now estimated at around 10^2 to 10^4 colony-forming units (CFU)/mL [3], with variations related to local pH, site of isolation, and environmental factors, such as food ingestion and medication intake. Furthermore, the pool of species and subspecies varies related to *H. pylori* status and related pathologic complications. Due to this multitude of factors, the differentiation

IntechOpen

between resident and transient microbiota and its role in health and disease remains controversial. Nevertheless, the potential of understanding the structure and dynamics of the gastric microbiota for the pathogenesis, diagnosis, and treatment of gastroduodenal diseases remains. Hence, this review aims to underline current knowledge on gastric microbiota and its relation to gastroduodenal pathology.

2. The hostile gastric environment

Compared to other gastrointestinal (GI) segments, the stomach has a physiological environment that is significantly more hostile to bacterial colonization and is a crucial part of the dynamics of the gastric microbiota. Primary reason for this is the gastric juice, which is composed of two main components—proteolytic enzymes and hydrochloric acid (HCl). The hydrochloric acid creates a strong acidic environment by maintaining a pH of 1–2 in the gastric lumen, which together with the proteolytic features of the gastric enzymes creates an intragastric environment that serves both digestive and protective roles. This environment facilitates the denaturation of proteins and nutrient absorption but also severely limits bacterial colonization and survival, preventing infection by pathogens [4]. The low pH value is the main restrictive component of the gastric juice [5]. To prevent damage to the mucosa from the acid and enzymes, neck cells of the gastric glands secrete mucus on the surface of the gastric epithelium. This mucus layer establishes a pH gradient that increases the pH up to 6–7 at the surface of the mucosa [6]. This is due to the unique properties of the mucus which permit acid to flow from parietal cells into crypts which communicate with the lumen, but do not allow acid at pH <4 from penetrating the mucus layer [6]. The mucus layer consists of several different mucin molecules, including MUC1, MUC5AC, MUC5AB, and MUC6, and forms two sublayers, an inner mucus layer that is firmly attached to the epithelia and a loose mucus layer, which is in direct contact with the lumen [7, 8]. Additional factors that contribute to the strong antimicrobial environment of the stomach are the accidental bile reflux and the gastric peristalsis.

3. *H. pylori*

In 1982 *Helicobacter pylori* was isolated by Barry Marshall and Robin Warren [1]. Their research changed the long-standing view that the stomach is as a sterile organ, being naturally hostile to bacterial survival. Today, it is known that *H. pylori* infects more than 50% of the world's population with the only significant reservoir for the infection appearing to be humans. Possible routes of infection include oral-oral, fecal-oral, and iatrogenic spread (e.g., by unsterile endoscopic interventions). In developing countries, infection is usually acquired early in childhood, unlike in industrialized countries, where it develops more commonly in adulthood [9].

H. pylori is a Gram-negative, spiral-shaped, motile, and flagellated bacteria that is uniquely adapted to colonizing the gastric niche. Hence, it comes with no surprise that when present, *H. pylori* has the highest relative abundance among all gastric microbial communities in both adults and children [10–12]. Upon infection, *H. pylori* utilizes urease and α-carbonic anhydrase to generate ammonia and HCO_3^-. This neutralizes H^+ and locally increases the pH, facilitating the bacteria's passage through the acidic gastric fluid and the pH-sensitive mucous layer. Using chemotaxis, the bacteria navigates the pH gradient to their niche near the host's epithelium [13, 14]. Once established in the inner mucus layer, *H. pylori* can utilize diverse adhesins (e.g., SabA and BabA) to attach to epithelial cells. Once attached, bacterial effector molecules, such as the vacuolating cytotoxin (VacA) and the cytotoxin-associated gene A (CagA), modulate the gastric epithelial cell behavior, leading to loss of cell polarity, release of nutrients and chemokines, and regulation of acid secretion via control of gastrin and H+/K+ ATPase [9, 15, 16]. In response to the *H. pylori* infection, the host mounts a complex inflammatory response, which ultimately leads to active chronic gastritis and subsequent gastroduodenal diseases. Therefore, the host's attempts to eradicate *H. pylori* increase gastric immunopathology (gastritis, epithelial damage such as atrophy and intestinal metaplasia), which alters the gastric compartment and its microbiota and may subsequently progress to gastric cancer.

4. Other non-*H. pylori* microbiota

4.1 Culture-dependent identification of gastric microbiota

Initial studies on the bacteria present in the stomach, using culture-based techniques, such as gastric juice cultures and mucosal biopsies were reported even before the isolation of *H. pylori*. In 1977 Savage DC [17] isolated bacteria from the stomach estimated at >10^3 CFU/g. The predominant phyla were *Firmicutes* (genera *Lactobacillus*, *Streptococcus*, *Clostridium*, and *Veillonella*), *Actinobacteria* (genus *Bifidobacterium*), and *Proteobacteria* (*coliforms*). However, due to the fact that these bacteria are prevalent along the whole GI tract, they were considered transient bacteria, which form small colonies that exist for short periods of time, rather than true gastric colonizers. Later culture-based studies [18–23] find that the most prevalent phylum, regardless of *H. pylori* status, is *Firmicutes*, followed by *Proteobacteria* and *Bacteroidetes*. *Actinobacteria* varies in studies as the second or third most prevalent phylum. The most commonly found genera were *Streptococcus*, *Lactobacillus*, *Bacteroides*, *Staphylococcus*, *Veillonella*, *Corynebacterium*, and *Neisseria*. However, given that culturing conditions for the majority of microbes colonizing the GI tract are not established, culture-based methods are considered to underestimate the gastric microbial diversity and are largely replaced by culture-independent methods.

4.2 Culture-independent identification of gastric microbiota

Culture-independent studies use a variety of molecular methods based on 16S rRNA gene sequencing. A multitude of reasons define these methods as far superior to those which are culture-dependent. These include:

- 16S rRNA is present in almost all bacteria.
- The function of the 16S rRNA gene has remained unchanged over time, suggesting that random sequence changes are a more accurate measure of time (evolution).
- The 16S rRNA gene is large enough for computational purposes [24].

A variety of 16S rRNA based methods exist, including:

- Fluorescent in situ hybridization (FISH) [25]
- Dot-blot hybridization with rRNA-targeted probes [26]
- Targeted qPCR [27]

- Traditional or sequence-aided community fingerprinting [28]
- Temperature gradient gel electrophoresis (TGGE) [29]
- Terminal restriction fragment length polymorphism (T-RFLP) [30]
- Sequencing of cloned 16S rDNA [29]
- Microarrays (PhyloChip) [31]
- Next-generation sequencing (NGS) [32]

In an extensive review of eight culture-independent studies, Sheh A. and Fox J. concluded that the most prominent phyla in the stomach are *Proteobacteria*, *Firmicutes*, *Bacteroidetes*, *Actinobacteria*, and *Fusobacteria* [33]. Furthermore, the most abundant phyla in *H. pylori*-positive subjects are *Proteobacteria*, *Firmicutes*, and *Actinobacteria*. In the absence of *H. pylori*, the most abundant phyla are *Firmicutes*, *Bacteroidetes*, and *Actinobacteria*. However, *H. pylori* remains the most dominant species in the stomach, comprising 72–99% of sequencing reads [10, 34]. In the absence of *H. pylori*, analysis consistently shows the presence of *Streptococcus* spp., which seem to be the most abundant genus in *H. pylori*-negative subjects [3, 30, 35, 36]. In the gastric microbiota, the non-*Helicobacter* genera commonly detected are *Streptococcus*, *Prevotella*, *Veillonella*, and *Rothia*.

5. Interrelations between *H. pylori* and other gastric microbiota

Numerous studies have shown significant variability of the gastric microbial communities with respect to *H. pylori* status. One such study was carried out by Osaki et al. [37], who examined the gastric microbiota of *H. pylori*-positive and *H. pylori*-negative Mongolian gerbils. The study showed a larger number of *Bifidobacterium* spp. in *H. pylori*-positive gerbils, compared to the *H. pylori*-negative, while *Eubacterium cylindroides* and *Prevotella* spp. were only found in the *H. pylori*-negative group.

Several mouse model studies have also shown clear differences in the composition of the gastric microbiota with respect to *H. pylori* status. Infection by *H. pylori* of pathogen-free female BALB/c mice has been shown to reduce the *Lactobacillus* spp. in the gastric microflora [26]. In transgenic, insulin-gastrin (INS-GAS) mice, the *H. pylori*-infected male mice show a significantly different phyla compared to the non-infected control group, with an increase in *Firmicutes* and a decrease in *Bacteroidetes* [26]. Findings in *H. pylori*-colonized C57BL/6 N female mice included reductions in *Firmicutes* (class *Bacilli*), *Bacteroidetes*, and *Proteobacteria* and an increase of *Firmicutes* (class *Clostridia*), *Proteobacteria* (genus *Helicobacter*), and *Verrucomicrobia*. However, other published data on the murine gastric microbiota suggest that neither acute nor chronic *H. pylori* infection substantially modifies the gastric microbial ecosystem [38].

A few studies have also examined *H. pylori*-related microbial differences in humans. One study found relative abundances of *Proteobacteria*, *Spirochetes*, and *Acidobacteria* in *H. pylori*-positive patients, compared to the control *H. pylori*-negative group. Another study demonstrated that patients positive for *H. pylori* culture showed significantly increased colonization of *Proteobacteria* and a decrease in *Actinobacteria* [39].

A few studies have given insight on how other microbial species can affect *H. pylori* by modulating *H. pylori*-induced gastric inflammatory responses. Two studies have indicated that the presence of intestinal *Helicobacter* (*H. bilis*, *H. hepaticus*, and *H. muridarum*) can both increase and decrease the severity of *H. pylori*-induced gastric inflammation by altering Treg cell responses [40, 41]. Another study demonstrated that *H. pylori* is present within the intestine in a coccoid form and that its interaction with phagocytes within the intestinal Peyer's patches modifies the intensity of *H. pylori*-induced gastritis [42]. However, other studies have shown that the gastric microbiota can accelerate gastric cancer progression in the presence of *H. pylori* and does so with no differences detected in the composition of the intestinal microbiota [27, 32].

As previously described *H. pylori* infection is associated with a multitude of changes in the gastric physiology and immunology, e.g., reduced gastric acidity, disturbed nutrient availability, and local inflammatory responses. These changes might be one explanation for the shift in the gastric microbial communities described, but the relation between *H. pylori* and non-*H. pylori* microbiota seems to be far more complex and remains to be further clarified. One problem is that so far, most studies are focused only on the effects of *H. pylori* on other microbiota, but little is known of how *H. pylori* is affected by other resident bacteria. Another problem is that different studies cannot be objectively compared, since they highly vary in methods and models used and the results depend on numerous other factors such as the time of *H. pylori* infection and the degree of mucosal inflammation. Therefore, further experiments are needed to give a more extensive understanding of these complex microbial interrelations.

6. Factors affecting the gastric microbiota

As described, *H. pylori* is the most significant species that colonizes the stomach and a key factor for the gastric microbial diversity but is far from sufficient to provide a wholesome understanding of the factors that determine its dynamics. Major factors that influence and define the dynamics of the gastric microbiota include gastric acidity, inflammation of the gastric mucosa, dietary habits, and use of medications.

6.1 Gastric acidity

The human gastric juice has an interprandial pH of between 1 and 2 in the gastric lumen, whereas with food ingestion it can reach up to pH 5. pH also varies in the different anatomical regions of the stomach, with most acidic being the fundus and the least being the antrum. The mucus lining the gastric mucosa establishes also a pH gradient from the lumen to the surface of the epithelium. This mucus consists of two sublayers—an inner mucus layer that is firmly attached to the epithelium and a variable mucus layer directly interacting with the lumen [7, 8]. Thus, across the mucus layer, the pH ranges from about 5.5 to 6.8 or even 7 at the surface of the gastric epithelial cells [5, 6]. It was already discussed that the low pH, caused by the hydrochloric acid, restricts the quantity of microorganisms and reduces the risk of infection by pathogens. Hence, sites with higher pH are significantly more hospitable to colonization and have a higher microbial density. Considerable fluctuations in the microbial density have been described with respect to the pH in the stomach, whereby both the quantity and the proportion of genera also fluctuate [43, 44]. Bacteria and bacterial DNA, which are isolated from gastric juice, differ from bacterial isolates adhering to the mucosa. During abnormal conditions, this balance may be different.

6.2 Dietary habits

While many studies document the effects of diet on the gut microbiota composition in humans, [45–49] there are only a few, mainly animal model studies, addressing the influence of diet on the gastric microbiota. An example is an in vivo study that compared the gastric microbiota of mice fed a non-purified diet (natural source-derived food) to mice fed a purified diet (refined food) and found higher levels of total aerobes, total anaerobes, and *Lactobacillus* in the stomach of the mice on a non-purified diet [50]. Nevertheless, it is well established how dietary factors affect the gastric microclimate, and since the microbiota is an inseparable part of this microclimate, it is not farfetched to suspect that diet affects the gastric microbial communities. However, more research is needed.

6.3 Use of medications

The long-term use of proton pump inhibitors (PPIs) and H2 antagonists affects the composition of the gastric microbiota by inducing a non-*H. pylori* bacterial overgrowth [51]. This is not surprising, considering that normally the non-*H. pylori* gastric microbiota is suppressed by the significantly acidic gastric environment. Suppression of gastric acidity will alter the bacterial flora of the upper GI tract, and studies have confirmed that PPIs do alter the bacterial population in the stomach [52]. This is mainly due to oral bacteria that survive instead of being killed in the normally acidic stomach. It has also been suspected that by causing alteration and overgrowth of the microbiota, acid-suppressive treatments may increase the risk of gastric cancer [52]. It has also been shown that a previously antrum-dominant *H. pylori* infection after treatment with acid inhibitors changed to a more corpus predominant infection [51]. The less acidic corpus allows *H. pylori* to penetrate deeper in the crypts and increase the inflammation, which causes faster progression to atrophy [53]. Treatment with acid inhibitors has by culture-dependent methods been shown to affect the survival of bacteria in the stomach. However, no significant differences have been found regarding diversity and composition of the microbiota by using culture methods [10].

Antibiotics are well known to have suppressive effects on the gastrointestinal microflora. *H. pylori* eradication is dependent on combined antibiotic treatment. However, certain antibiotic treatments can have negative effects on the "healthy" gastric microbiota. Animal studies indicate that treatment with penicillins reduces *Lactobacillus* populations and promotes yeast colonization of the gastric epithelium. Furthermore, Mason et al. [54] showed that cefoperazone treatment in humans causes long-term alteration of the gastric microbiota, such as a significant reduction in the number of *Lactobacillus* and overgrowth of *Enterococcus*.

7. Gastric microbiota and gastroduodenal diseases

7.1 Chronic gastritis and peptic ulcer disease

The isolation of *H. pylori* was a real breakthrough, not because it declared the stomach as a non-sterile organ but because subsequent research established it as a main etiological factor for the development of gastroduodenal diseases [2, 55, 56]. It is well known that long-term *H. pylori* infection causes various degrees of chronic inflammation of the underlying gastric mucosa. A subset of patients develops clinical symptoms, and a further subset will develop complications including peptic ulcer, gastric mucosa-associated lymphoid tissue (MALT) lymphoma, and gastric cancer. The cascade leading from chronic gastritis to neoplasm is known as Correa's cascade and involves the progression to glandular atrophy with intestinal metaplasia and dysplasia and eventually to invasive carcinoma [57]. Peptic ulcer disease is the most common complication of chronic *H. pylori* infection, with 95% of duodenal and 70% of gastric ulcers being linked to it [58]. All of this serves to prove that *H. pylori* is by far the most important microbial species that can colonize the stomach, with an enormous impact on the pathogenesis and development of gastroduodenal diseases.

Nevertheless, there is arising evidence that non-*H. pylori* bacteria may also play an important role in the pathogenesis of chronic gastritis and peptic ulcers. One study suggests that different gastric microbial communities, such as the overrepresentation of the *Streptococcus* genus within the *Firmicutes* phylum, can lead to gastritis as well, even in the absence of *H. pylori* [35]. Another study has found an increase of *Streptococcus* and a decrease of *Prevotella* in patients with atrophic gastritis, versus healthy subjects [59]. There are also several studies that assess the role of non-*H. pylori* species in peptic ulcer disease. The non-*H. pylori* bacteria seems to be more prevalent in patients with non-ulcer dyspepsia than in those with gastric ulcer as shown by a culture-based study by Hu et al. [19]. Another study in Malaysian patients showed significant correlation between the isolation of *Streptococcus* and patients with peptic ulcers [60]. Given that most studies find that the *Streptococcus* genus is one of the most abundant non-*H. pylori* species in the stomach, a possible pathogenic relation can be a subject of further research. However, by far no other species have an established pathogenic role except *H. pylori*.

7.2 Gastric cancer

Each year approximately 990,000 people are diagnosed with gastric cancer (GC) worldwide, of whom about 738,000 die from this disease, making GC the fourth most common incident cancer and the second most common cause of cancer death. Both incidence and mortality rates are about twice as high in males as in females. Over 70% of cases occur in developing nations, concentrated in Eastern Asia, Eastern Europe, and Central and South America. Approximately 90% of gastric cancers are adenocarcinomas, with the other 10% shared between mucosa-associated lymphoid tissue (MALT) lymphomas, gastrointestinal stromal tumors (GIST), leiomyosarcomas, and other more rare types of cancer. Adenocarcinomas are histologically classified into two major types: diffuse and intestinal. These two types not only look different under the microscope but also differ in gender ratio, age at diagnosis, and other epidemiologic features. Anatomically, gastric cancers are categorized as proximal and distal. Proximal adenocarcinomas are more similar to esophageal adenocarcinomas and may be associated with the absence of *H. pylori*, while distal adenocarcinomas originate in the antrum, with approximately 90% of such cases related to *H. pylori* infection [61]. Today the correlation between *H. pylori* and the development of gastric cancer is undeniable as shown in several prospective studies [62–64]. Moreover, the eradication of *H. pylori* is proven to significantly reduce the risk of gastric cancer development, according to several international consensuses [65, 66]. *H. pylori* was recognized as a “definite carcinogen” by the World Health Organization in 1994, and this fact was reconfirmed in 2009.

However, *H. pylori* coevolved with humans for millennia, and only 1–2% of people infected with this bacterium actually develop gastric cancer or MALT lymphoma. Similar to most cancers, pathogenetic mechanisms remain unclear with a multitude of other factors to influence the final carcinogenesis [61]. Although, *H. pylori* is clearly the most relevant microbial risk factor for the development of gastric cancer, an increasing pool of evidence suggests that other microbial communities play a causative role in the pathophysiology of gastric cancer. To date, several animal and human studies have supported this theory.

Studies with INS-GAS mice have revealed that male mice with intestinal microbiota developed gastric pathology from chronic gastritis to atrophy and dysplasia independent of *H. pylori* infection. Furthermore, the presence of commensal microbiota accelerated the progression to gastric intraepithelial neoplasia, and gastric intraepithelial neoplasia became invasive in *H. pylori*-infected INS-GAS mice. Male INS-GAS mice with *H. pylori* infection, colonized with artificial mouse intestinal microbiota, have shown increased incidence of gastric intraepithelial neoplasia by 69% [27, 32]. On the other hand, antibiotic treatments significantly delayed the onset of gastric neoplasia in *Helicobacter*-free and specific pathogen-free INS-GAS mice [67].

A study by Wang et al. found a similar number of bacterial species in the microbiota between gastric cancer and chronic gastritis, but by using a method to explore and visualize similarities or dissimilarities of the data, a pattern suggesting the presence of a diversified microbiota in gastric cancer was found [68]. Moreover, a 16S rRNA gene sequencing analysis of gastric mucosa of patients with gastric cancer showed a prevalence of the genera *Lactobacillus*, *Streptococcus* (among which the most common species were *S. mitis* and *Streptococcus parasanguinis*), *Prevotella*, and *Veillonella* [30]. Two other studies evaluated the gastric microbiota of subjects with non-atrophic gastritis, intestinal metaplasia, and gastric cancer. The first one showed a significantly lower diversity and a higher abundance of the genus *Pseudomonas* in the microbiota of neoplastic patients compared to patients with simple gastritis. Moreover, both the progressive decrease of six taxa and the progressive increase of two taxa were observed from the gastritis group to the neoplastic group, via the metaplastic group [69]. In the second study, a high-throughput sequencing platform was used for the assessment of gastric microbiota in the three groups, showing definitely different results: a greater bacterial diversity, a relative rise of *Bacilli* and *Streptococcaceae*, and a relative reduction of *Helicobacteraceae* were found in the cancer group compared to other groups [70].

It is possible that non-*H. pylori* species potentiate carcinogenesis through various mechanisms, such as promoting inflammation, stimulating cell proliferation, modifying stem cell dynamics, and producing toxic metabolites [71]. However, it is still unsure whether the different microbial structure is causative for the carcinogenesis or carcinogenesis itself causes a shift in the microbial communities, which subsequently promotes carcinogenesis further.

8. Gastric microbiota and extra-gastric diseases

The stomach is part of the GI tract, and as such, possible relations between the gastric microbiota's composition and diseases of other parts of the GI tract, such as the esophagus (esophagitis and esophageal cancer), small intestines, and colon cannot be overlooked [72]. One study, using 16S rDNA analyses of duodenal aspirates, demonstrated lower diversity in irritable bowel syndrome patients compared to controls with significant alterations in 12 genera [73]. An increased risk for colorectal neoplasia in *H. pylori*-infected patients has been confirmed by many large-scale studies [74, 75].

Other studies have addressed the association between autoimmune hepatitis and altered microbiome of the upper GI tract and found this to be linked to increased intestinal permeability [76].

Regarding the extra-gastrointestinal involvement of gastric microbiota (especially *H. pylori*), studies find possible associations with hematological diseases like idiopathic thrombocytopenic purpura [77] and anemia [78] and cardiovascular [79], neurological [80], and endocrine [81] diseases.

Nevertheless, research in this field is far from sufficient to be conclusive.

9. Discussion

It is undeniable that *H. pylori* is by far the most unique and important species that can colonize the gastric niche with clear pathogenic significance to

DOI: http://dx.doi.org/10.5772/intechopen.86926

gastroduodenal diseases. However, culture-dependent and later culture-independent studies prove that the stomach harbors a complex microbiota with many other phyla (*Proteobacteria*, *Firmicutes*, *Bacteroidetes*, *Actinobacteria*, and *Fusobacteria*) and genera (*Lactobacillus*, *Streptococcus*, *Clostridium*, *Prevotella*, *Veillonella*, *Bifidobacterium*, and *Rothia*) being identified. By far, it is arguable which genera can be considered resident since results depend on a multitude of factors, among which gastric acidity stands out as the most significant. However, it is worth noting that *Streptococcus*, *Prevotella*, *Veillonella*, and *Rothia* seem to be the most abundant genera in *H. pylori*-negative subjects. Nevertheless, the significance of both transient and resident non-*H. pylori* microbiota lies in its possible role in the development and progression of gastroduodenal diseases, such as gastritis, peptic ulcer disease, and gastric cancer. So far, only a few and far from enough studies suggest that non-*H. pylori* microbiota can lead to gastric pathology in the absence of *H. pylori*. However, findings are convincing that the non-*H. pylori* microbiota can play an important role in modulating *H. pylori*-induced gastric inflammation, influencing an individual's risk of gastric diseases and consequently the severity of the resulting disease. Suspected pathophysiologic mechanisms involved in this include modulating immune cell responses, stimulating cell proliferation, modifying stem cell dynamics, and producing toxic metabolites. Although, substantial advancements in unrevealing the complexity of the gastric microbiota and its' role in health and disease have been made, studies are far from sufficient to suggest new strategies for prevention, diagnosis, and treatment of gastroduodenal diseases. However, this potential remains and undoubtedly should be further explored.

Acknowledgements

The publication of this work was supported by KRKA.

Conflict of interest

There are no conflicts of interest.

Author details

Hristo Ilianov Iliev[1*], Mila Dimitrova Kovacheva-Slavova[2], Todor Asenov Angelov[2], Hristo Yankov Valkov[2], Ali Bedran[3] and Borislav Georgiev Vladimirov[2]

1 Medical University—Sofia, Sofia, Bulgaria

2 Department of Gastroenterology, University Hospital "Tsaritsa Ioanna-ISUL", Medical University of Sofia, Sofia, Bulgaria

3 Clinical Laboratory, University Hospital "Tsaritsa Ioanna-ISUL", Sofia, Bulgaria, Medical University of Sofia, Sofia, Bulgaria

*Address all correspondence to: hilievbg@gmail.com

References

[1] Warren JR, Marshall BJ. Unidentified curved bacilli on gastric epithelium in active chronic gastritis. Lancet. 1983;**1**:1273-1275. DOI: 10.1016/S0140-6736(83)92719-8

[2] Wang F, Meng W, Wang B, Qiao L. *Helicobacter pylori*-induced gastric inflammation and gastric cancer. Cancer Letters. 2014;**345**(2):196-202. DOI: 10.1016/j.canlet.2013.08.016

[3] Delgado S, Cabrera-Rubio R, Mira A, Suárez A, Mayo B. Microbiological survey of the human gastric ecosystem using culturing and pyrosequencing methods. Microbial Ecology. 2013;**65**(3):763-772. DOI: 10.1007/s00248-013-0192-5

[4] Martinsen TC, Bergh K, Waldum HL. Gastric juice: A barrier against infectious diseases. Basic & Clinical Pharmacology & Toxicology. 2005;**96**:94-102. DOI: 10.1111/j.1742-7843.2005.pto960202.x

[5] Manson JM, Rauch M, Gilmore MS. The commensal microbiology of the gastrointestinal tract. Advances in Experimental Medicine and Biology. 2008;**635**:15-28. DOI: 10.1007/978-0-387-09550-9_2

[6] Bhaskar KR, Garik P, Turner BS, Bradley JD, Bansil R, Stanley HE, et al. Viscous fingering of HCl through gastric mucin. Nature. 1992;**360**:458-461. DOI: 10.1038/360458a0

[7] Corfield AP, Carroll D, Myerscough N, Probert CS. Mucins in the gastrointestinal tract in health and disease. Frontiers in Bioscience. 2001;**6**:D1321-D1357. DOI: 10.2741/Corfield

[8] Atuma C, Strugala V, Allen A, Holm L. The adherent gastrointestinal mucus gel layer: Thickness and physical state in vivo. American Journal of Physiology. Gastrointestinal and Liver Physiology. 2001;**280**:G922-G929. DOI: 10.1152/ajpgi.2001.280.5.G922

[9] Kusters JG, van Vliet AH, Kuipers EJ. Pathogenesis of *Helicobacter pylori* infection. Clinical Microbiology Reviews. 2006;**19**(3):449-490. DOI: 10.1128/CMR.00054-05

[10] Bik EM, Eckburg PB, Gill SR, et al. Molecular analysis of the bacterial microbiota in the human stomach. Proceedings of the National Academy of Sciences of the United States of America. 2006;**103**(3):732-737. DOI: 10.1073/pnas.0506655103

[11] Schulz C, Schütte K, Koch N, et al. The active bacterial assemblages of the upper GI tract in individuals with and without *Helicobacter* infection. Gut. 2016;**67**(2):216-225. DOI: 10.1136/gutjnl-2016-312904

[12] Llorca L, Pérez-Pérez G, Urruzuno P, et al. Characterization of the gastric microbiota in a pediatric population according to *Helicobacter pylori* status. The Pediatric Infectious Disease Journal. 2017;**36**(2):173-178. DOI: 10.1097/INF.0000000000001383

[13] Williams SM, Chen YT, Andermann TM, Carter JE, McGee DJ, Ottemann KM. *Helicobacter pylori* chemotaxis modulates inflammation and bacterium-gastric epithelium interactions in infected mice. Infection and Immunity. 2007;**75**:3747-3757. DOI: 10.1128/IAI.00082-07

[14] Croxen MA, Sisson G, Melano R, Hoffman PS. The *Helicobacter pylori* chemotaxis receptor TlpB (HP0103) is required for pH taxis and for colonization of the gastric mucosa. Journal of Bacteriology. 2006;**188**:2656-2665. DOI: 10.1128/JB.188.7.2656-2665.2006

[15] Saha A, Backert S, Hammond CE, Gooz M, Smolka AJ. *Helicobacter pylori* CagL activates ADAM17 to induce repression of the gastric H, K-ATPase alpha subunit. Gastroenterology. 2010;**139**:239-248. DOI: 10.1053/j.gastro.2010.03.036

[16] O'Keeffe J, Moran AP. Conventional, regulatory, and unconventional T cells in the immunologic response to *Helicobacter pylori*. Helicobacter. 2008;**13**:1-19. DOI: 10.1111/j.1523-5378.2008.00559.x

[17] Savage DC. Microbial ecology of the gastrointestinal tract. Annual Review of Microbiology. 1977;**31**:107-133. DOI: 10.1146/annurev.mi.31.100177.000543

[18] Stockbruegger RW. Bacterial overgrowth as a consequence of reduced gastric acidity. Scandinavian Journal of Gastroenterology. Supplement. 1985;**111**:7-16. DOI: 10.3109/00365528509093749

[19] Hu Y, He LH, Xiao D, Liu GD, Gu YX, Tao XX, et al. Bacterial flora concurrent with *Helicobacter pylori* in the stomach of patients with upper gastrointestinal diseases. World Journal of Gastroenterology. 2012;**18**:1257-1261. DOI: 10.3748/wjg.v18.i11.1257

[20] Zilberstein B, Quintanilha AG, Santos MA, Pajecki D, Moura EG, Alves PR, et al. Clinics (São Paulo, Brazil). 2007;**62**:47-54. DOI: 10.1590/S1807-59322007000100008

[21] Sharma BK, Santana IA, Wood EC, Walt RP, Pereira M, Noone P, et al. Intragastric bacterial activity and nitrosation before, during, and after treatment with omeprazole. British Medical Journal. 1984;**289**:717-719. DOI: 10.1136/bmj.289.6447.717

[22] Adamsson I, Nord CE, Lundquist P, Sjöstedt S, Edlund C. Comparative effects of omeprazole, amoxycillin plus metronidazole versus omeprazole, clarithromycin plus metronidazole on the oral, gastric and intestinal microflora in *Helicobacter pylori*-infected patients. The Journal of Antimicrobial Chemotherapy. 1999;**44**:629-640. DOI: 10.1093/jac/44.5.629

[23] Sjöstedt S, Heimdahl A, Kager L, Nord CE. Microbial colonization of the oropharynx, esophagus and stomach in patients with gastric diseases. European Journal of Clinical Microbiology. 1985;**4**:49-51. DOI: 10.1007/BF02148660

[24] Janda JM, Abbott SL. 16S rRNA gene sequencing for bacterial identification in the diagnostic laboratory: Pluses, perils, and pitfalls. Journal of Clinical Microbiology. 2007;**45**(9):2761-2764. DOI: 10.1128/JCM.01228-07

[25] Langendijk PS, Schut F, Jansen GJ, Raangs GC, Kamphuis GR, Wilkinson MH, et al. Quantitative fluorescence in situ hybridization of *Bifidobacterium* spp. with genus-specific 16S rRNAtargeted probes and its application in fecal samples. Applied and Environmental Microbiology. 1995;**61**:3069-3075

[26] Aebischer T, Fischer A, Walduck A, Schlötelburg C, Lindig M, Schreiber S, et al. Vaccination prevents *Helicobacter pylori*-induced alterations of the gastric flora in mice. FEMS Immunology and Medical Microbiology. 2006;**46**: 221-229. DOI: 10.1111/rp10.1016-j.femsim.2004.05.008

[27] Lertpiriyapong K, Whary MT, Muthupalani S, Lofgren JL, Gamazon ER, Feng Y, et al. Gastric colonisation with a restricted commensal microbiota replicates the promotion of neoplastic lesions by diverse intestinal microbiota in the *Helicobacter pylori* INS-GAS mouse model of gastric carcinogenesis. Gut. 2013;**63**:54-63. DOI: 10.1136/gutjnl-2013-305178

[28] Heilig HG, Zoetendal EG, Vaughan EE, Marteau P, Akkermans AD,

de Vos WM. Molecular diversity of *Lactobacillus* spp. and other lactic acid bacteria in the human intestine as determined by specific amplification of 16S ribosomal DNA. Applied and Environmental Microbiology. 2002;**68**:114-123. DOI: 10.1128/AEM.68.1.114-123.2002

[29] Monstein HJ, Tiveljung A, Kraft CH, Borch K, Jonasson J. Profiling of bacterial flora in gastric biopsies from patients with *Helicobacter pylori*-associated gastritis and histologically normal control individuals by temperature gradient gel electrophoresis and 16SrDNA sequence analysis. Journal of Medical Microbiology. 2000;**49**:817-822. DOI: 10.1099/0022-1317-49-9-817

[30] Dicksved J, Lindberg M, Rosenquist M, Enroth H, Jansson JK, Engstrand L. Molecular characterization of the stomach microbiota in patients with gastric cancer and in controls. Journal of Medical Microbiology. 2009;**58**:509-516. DOI: 10.1099/jmm.0.007302-0

[31] Rolig AS, Cech C, Ahler E, Carter JE, Ottemann KM. The degree of *Helicobacter pylori*-triggered inflammation is manipulated by preinfection host microbiota. Infection and Immunity. 2013;**81**:1382-1389. DOI: 10.1128/IAI.00044-13

[32] Lofgren JL, Whary MT, Ge Z, Muthupalani S, et al. Lack of commensal flora in *Helicobacter pylori*-infected INS-GAS mice reduces gastritis and delays intraepithelial neoplasia. Gastroenterology. 2011;**140**:210-220. DOI: 10.1053/j.gastro.2010.09.048

[33] Sheh A, Fox JG. The role of the gastrointestinal microbiome in *Helicobacter pylori* pathogenesis. Gut Microbes. 2013;**4**(6):505-531. DOI: 10.4161/gmic.26205

[34] Andersson AF, Lindberg M, Jakobsson H, Bäckhed F, Nyrén P, Engstrand L. Comparative analysis of human gut microbiota by barcoded pyrosequencing. PLoS One. 2008;**3**:e2836. DOI: 10.1371/journal.pone.0002836

[35] Li XX, Wong GL, To KF, Wong VW, Lai LH, Chow DK, et al. Bacterial microbiota profiling in gastritis without *Helicobacter pylori* infection or non-steroidal anti-inflammatory drug use. PLoS One. 2009;**4**:e7985. DOI: 10.1371/journal.pone.0007985

[36] Stearns JC, Lynch MD, Senadheera DB, Tenenbaum HC, Goldberg MB, Cvitkovitch DG, et al. Bacterial biogeography of the human digestive tract. Scientific Reports. 2011;**1**:170. DOI: 10.1038/srep00170

[37] Osaki T, Matsuki T, Asahara T, Zaman C, Hanawa T, Yonezawa H, et al. Comparative analysis of gastric bacterial microbiota in Mongolian gerbils after long-term infection with *Helicobacter pylori*. Microbial Pathogenesis. 2012;**53**(1):12-18

[38] Tan MP, Kaparakis M, Galic M, Pedersen J, Pearse M, Wijburg OL, et al. Chronic *Helicobacter pylori* infection does dot significantly alter the microbiota of the murine stomach. Applied and Environmental Microbiology. 2007;**73**(3):1010-1013

[39] Maldonado-Contreras A, Goldfarb KC, Godoy-Vitorino F, et al. Structure of the human gastric bacterial community in relation to *Helicobacter pylori* status. The ISME Journal. 2010;**5**(4):574-579. DOI: 10.1038/ismej.2010.149

[40] Lemke LB, Ge Z, Whary MT, et al. Concurrent *Helicobacter bilis* infection in C57BL/6 mice attenuates proinflammatory *H. pylori*-induced gastric pathology. Infection and Immunity. 2009;**77**(5):2147-2158. DOI: 10.1128/IAI.01395-08

[41] Ge Z, Feng Y, Muthupalani S, et al. Infection and Immunity.

2011;**79**(10):3861-3871. DOI: 10.1128/IAI.05357-11

[42] Nagai S, Mimuro H, Yamada T, et al. Role of Peyer's patches in the induction of *Helicobacter pylori*-induced gastritis. Proceedings of the National Academy of Sciences of the United States of America. 2007;**104**(21):8971-8976. DOI: 10.1073/pnas.0609014104

[43] Draser BS, Shiner M, McLeod GM. Studies of the intestinal flora 1. The bacterial flora of the gastrointestinal tract in healthy and achlorhydric patients. Gastroenterology. 1969;**56**:71-79

[44] Milton-Thompson GJ, Lightfoot NF, Ahmet Z, et al. Intragastric acidity, bacteria, nitrite, and N-nitroso compounds before, during, and after cimetidine treatment. Lancet. 1982;**1**(8281):1091-1095

[45] Goldsmith JR, Sartor RB. The role of diet on intestinal microbiota metabolism: Downstream impacts on host immune function and health, and therapeutic implications. Journal of Gastroenterology. 2014;**49**(5):785-798. DOI: 10.1007/s00535-014-0953-z

[46] Korpela K, Flint HJ, Johnstone AM, et al. Gut microbiota signatures predict host and microbiota responses to dietary interventions in obese individuals. PLoS One. 2014;**9**(6):e90702. DOI: 10.1371/journal.pone.0090702

[47] David LA, Maurice CF, Carmody RN, et al. Diet rapidly and reproducibly alters the human gut microbiome. Nature. 2013;**505**(7484):559-563. DOI: 10.1038/nature12820

[48] Chan YK, Estaki M, Gibson DL. Clinical consequences of diet-induced dysbiosis. Annals of Nutrition and Metabolism. 2013;**63**(suppl 2):28-40. DOI: 10.1159/000354902

[49] Fan W, Huo G, Li X, et al. Impact of diet in shaping gut microbiota revealed by a comparative study in infants during the six months of life. Journal of Microbiology and Biotechnology. 2014;**24**(2):133-143

[50] Wu GD, Chen J, Hoffmann C, et al. Linking long-term dietary patterns with gut microbial enterotypes. Science. 2011;**334**:105-108. DOI: 10.1126/science.1208344

[51] Sanduleanu S, Jonkers D, De Bruine A, Hameeteman W, Stockbrügger RW. Non-*Helicobacter pylori* bacterial flora during acid-suppressive therapy: Differential findings in gastric juice and gastric mucosa. Alimentary Pharmacology & Therapeutics. 2001;**15**(3):379-388. DOI: 10.1046/j.1365-2036.2001.00888.x

[52] Williams C, McColl KEL. Review article: Proton pump inhibitors and bacterial overgrowth. Alimentary Pharmacology & Therapeutics. 2006;**23**(1):3-10. DOI: 10.1111/j.1365-2036.2006.02707.x

[53] Meuwissen SG, Craanen ME, Kuipers EJ. Gastric mucosal morphological consequences of acid suppression: A balanced view. Best practice & research. Clinical Gastroenterology. 2001;**15**(3):497-510. DOI: 10.1053/bega.2001.0189

[54] Mason KL, Erb Downward JR, Falkowski NR, Young VB, Kao JY, Huffnagle GB. Interplay between the gastric bacterial microbiota and *Candida albicans* during postantibiotic recolonization and gastritis. Infection and Immunity. 2012;**80**(1):150-158. DOI: 10.1128/IAI.05162-11

[55] Zhang X, Zhang J, Lin Y, Xu K, Li N, Chen H, et al. Analysis of the relationship between invasive capability of *Helicobacter pylori* and gastroduodenal diseases. Journal of Medical Microbiology. 2015

May;**64**(Pt 5):498-506. DOI: 10.1099/jmm.0.000049

[56] Blaser MJ, Atherton JC. *Helicobacter pylori* persistence: Biology and disease. The Journal of Clinical Investigation. 2004;**113**(3):321-333. DOI: 10.1172/JCI20925

[57] Correa P, Piazuelo MB. *Helicobacter pylori* infection and gastric adenocarcinoma. US Gastroenterology and Hepatology Review. 2011;**7**(1):59-64

[58] Ford AC, Gurusamy KS, Delaney B, Forman D, Moayyedi P. Eradication therapy for peptic ulcer disease in *Helicobacter pylori*-positive people. Cochrane Database of Systematic Reviews. 2016;**4**:CD003840. DOI: 10.1002/14651858.CD003840.pub5

[59] Engstrand L, Lindberg M. *Helicobacter pylori* and the gastric microbiota. Best Practice & Research. Clinical Gastroenterology. 2013;**27**: 39-45. DOI: 10.1016/j.bpg.2013.03.016

[60] Khosravi Y, Dieye Y, Poh BH, et al. Culturable bacterial microbiota of the stomach of *Helicobacter pylori* positive and negative gastric disease patients. The Scientific World Journal. 2014;**2014**:610421. DOI: 10.1155/2014/610421

[61] Karimi P, Islami F, Anandasabapathy S, Freedman ND, Kamangar F. Gastric cancer: Descriptive epidemiology, risk factors, screening, and prevention. Cancer Epidemiology, Biomarkers & Prevention. 2014;**23**(5):700-713. DOI: 10.1158/1055-9965.EPI-13-1057

[62] Forman D, Newell DG, Fullerton F, et al. Association between infection with *Helicobacter pylori* and risk of gastric cancer: Evidence from a prospective investigation. BMJ. 1991;**302**(6788):1302-1305

[63] Nomura A, Stemmermann GN, Chyou PH, Kato I, Perez-Perez GI, Blaser MJ. *Helicobacter pylori* infection and gastric carcinoma among Japanese Americans in Hawaii. The New England Journal of Medicine. 1991;**325**(16):1132-1136. DOI: 10.1056/NEJM199110173251604

[64] Hsu PI, Lai KH, Hsu PN, et al. *Helicobacter pylori* infection and the risk of gastric malignancy. The American Journal of Gastroenterology. 2007;**102**(4):725-730. DOI: 10.1111/j.1572-0241.2006.01109.x

[65] Malfertheiner P, Megraud F, O'Morain CA, et al. Management of *Helicobacter pylori* infection--the Maastricht IV/ Florence consensus report. Gut. 2012;**61**(5):646-664. DOI: 10.1136/gutjnl-2012-302084

[66] Sheu BS, Wu MS, Chiu CT, et al. Consensus on the clinical management, screening-to-treat, and surveillance of *Helicobacter pylori* infection to improve gastric cancer control on a nationwide scale. Helicobacter. 2017;**22**(3):e12368. DOI: 10.1111/hel.12368

[67] Lee CW, Rickman B, Rogers AB, et al. Combination of sulindac and antimicrobial eradication of *Helicobacter pylori* prevents progression of gastric cancer in hypergastrinemic INS-GAS mice. Cancer Research. 2009;**69**(20):8166-8174. DOI: 10.1158/0008-5472.CAN-08-3856

[68] Wang L, Zhou J, Xin Y, Geng C, Tian Z, Yu X, et al. Bacterial overgrowth and diversification of microbiota in gastric cancer. European Journal of Gastroenterology & Hepatology. 2016;**28**(3):261-266. DOI: 10.1097/MEG.0000000000000542

[69] Eun CS, Kim BK, Han DS, Kim SY, Kim KM, Choi BY, et al. Differences in gastric mucosal microbiota profiling in patients with chronic gastritis, intestinal metaplasia, and gastric cancer using

pyrosequencing methods. Helicobacter. 2014;**19**:407-416. DOI: 10.1111/hel.12145

[70] Walker MM, Talley NJ. Review article: Bacteria and pathogenesis of disease in the upper gastrointestinal tract–beyond the era of *Helicobacter pylori*. Alimentary Pharmacology & Therapeutics. 2014;**39**(8):767-779. DOI: 10.1111/apt.12666

[71] Alarcon T, Lorca L, Pereze-Perez G. Impact of microbiota and gastric disease development by *Helicobacter pylori*. Current Topics in Microbiology and Immunology. 2017;**400**:253-275. DOI: 10.1007/978-3-319-50520-6_11

[72] Ianiro G, Molina-Infante J, Gasbarrini A. Gastric microbiota. Helicobacter. 2015;**20**(Suppl. 1):68-71. DOI: 10.1111/hel.12260

[73] Giamarellos-Bourboulis E, Tang J, Pyleris E, Pistiki A, Barbatzas C, Brown J, et al. Molecular assessment of differences in the duodenal microbiome in subjects with irritable bowel syndrome. Scandinavian Journal of Gastroenterology. 2015;**50**(9):1076-1087. DOI: 10.3109/00365521.2015.1027261

[74] Zhang Y, Hoffmeister M, Weck MN, Chang-Claude J, Brenner H. *Helicobacter pylori* infection and colorectal cancer risk: Evidence from a large population-based case-control study in Germany. American Journal of Epidemiology. 2012;**175**(5):441-450. DOI: 10.1093/aje/kwr331

[75] Kim TJ, Kim ER, Chang DK, et al. *Helicobacter pylori* infection is an independent risk factor of early and advanced colorectal neoplasm. Helicobacter. 2017;**22**(3):e12377. DOI: 10.1111/hel.12377

[76] Lin R, Zhou L, Zhang J, Wang B. Abnormal intestinal permeability and microbiota in patients with autoimmune hepatitis. International Journal of Clinical and Experimental Pathology. 2015;**8**(5):5153-5160

[77] Franchini M, Vescovi PP, Garofano M, Veneri D. *Helicobacter pylori*-associated idiopathic thrombocytopenic purpura: A narrative review. Seminars in Thrombosis and Hemostasis. 2012;**38**(5):463-468. DOI: 10.1055/s-0032-1305781

[78] Cardenas VM, Mulla ZD, Ortiz M, Graham DY. Iron deficiency and *Helicobacter pylori* infection in the United States. American Journal of Epidemiology. 2006;**163**(2):127-134. DOI: 10.1093/aje/kwj018

[79] Nam SY, Park BJ, Ryu KH, Nam JH. Effect of *Helicobacter pylori* eradication on the regression of gastric polyps in National Cancer Screening Program. The Korean Journal of Internal Medicine. 2017;**33**(3):506-511. DOI: 10.3904/kjim.2016.286

[80] Suwarnalata G, Tan AH, Isa H, et al. Augmentation of autoantibodies by *Helicobacter pylori* in Parkinson's disease patients may be linked to greater severity. PLoS One. 2016;**11**(4):e0153725. DOI: 10.1371/journal.pone.0153725

[81] Wang F, Liu J, Lv Z. Association of *Helicobacter pylori* infection with diabetes mellitus and diabetic nephropathy: A meta-analysis of 39 studies involving more than 20,000 participants. Scandinavian Journal of Infectious Diseases. 2013;**45**(12):930-938. DOI: 10.3109/00365548.2013.844351

Section 2

Stomas Prevention

Chapter 5

Full Colonoscopy in Patients under 50 Years Old with Lower Gastrointestinal Bleeding

Mahsa Khodadoostan, Ahmad Shavakhi,
Reihaneh Padidarnia, Alireza Shavakhi and Mehdi Ahmadian

Abstract

The aim of this study is to compare sigmoidoscopy with full colonoscopy in these patients. In this cross-sectional study, 120 eligible patients under 50 years old with acute rectal bleeding were enrolled. Pain, the comfort of the test by physician and patient, duration of the procedure, and pathologic findings were recorded during sigmoidoscopy and proximal colonoscopy (from splenic flexure to ileocecal valve) in the same patient. The variables in the two stages were compared with each other. There were 66 women (55%) and 54 men (45%), and the mean of age was 41 ± 7.9 years. Proximal colonoscopy from splenic flexure to reach cecum was relatively easier for the physician and the patient than sigmoidoscopy ($P < 0.001$). Furthermore, the time spent to carry out proximal colonoscopy was less than the time taken for sigmoidoscopy ($P < 0.001$). Pathologic findings recorded in full colonoscopy were more than sigmoidoscopy ($P < 0.001$). Therefore, full colonoscopy that includes sigmoidoscopy and proximal colonoscopy is relatively easier than sigmoidoscopy for patients, and it also proves to be more advantageous than sigmoidoscopy for physicians to perform in Iranian patients because of the more tortuous and elongated sigmoid colon in these patients.

Keywords: colonoscopy, gastrointestinal bleeding, sigmoidoscopy

1. Introduction

Lower gastrointestinal bleeding (LGIB) is one of the most common problems that gastroenterologists and surgeons encountered [1]. LGIB prevalence increases with aging, using aspirin, anticoagulants, and nonsteroidal anti-inflammatory drugs (NASIDs). LGIB is associated with death, hospitalization, and medical costs [2]. Therefore, diagnosis of the cause of LGIB and its proper management are of critical importance [3]. These causes include bleeding from the diverticulum, ischemic colitis, angiodysplasia, hemorrhoids, colorectal cancer, inflammatory bowel disease, infectious colitis, NSAID, radiation, and solitary ulcers [4, 5]. For diagnosing the causes of lower bleeding (LGIB), there are different modalities such as total colonoscopy, radionuclide scan, angiography, computed tomography angiography, and sigmoidoscopy [6].

Some authors believe that in 90% of patients <50 years who present with LGIB, most causes are benign anorectal diseases, and on the other hand, the prevalence of colorectal cancer increases with aging. Hence, patients <50 years who present with LGIB are examined excessively in whom there is no need for total colonoscopy and sigmoidoscopy alone is enough [7, 8]. In some researches, it is expressed that total examination of the colon in these individuals through total colonoscopy will impose stress on them and longer hospitalization [9]. On the other hand, some researchers believe that colonoscopy should be applied on all individuals who present with LGIB for its high authority in diagnosing other damages such as polyp and colorectal cancers [10]. Furthermore, they believe that in patients who were under sigmoidoscopy, performing colonoscopy is causing more diagnosing dangerous and deadly diseases through neoplasms, but, in total colonoscopy, it is required for complete preparation and totally clean intestines which may impose strong pain. In some circumstances, there arises the need for using anesthetics and longtime hospitalization [11]. Currently, there is no any definite consensus about whether the patients with LGIB would be under total colonoscopy or only sigmoidoscopy can be enough. The purpose of this study is to analyze and compare the methods of colonoscopy and sigmoidoscopy regarding the additional findings and easiness of them for patients and physician in patients <50 years with LGIB.

In this cross-sectional study performed from January 2016 to November 2016 in Al-Zahra Hospital in Isfahan, 120 patients with LGIB were referred, and informed consent for participation was obtained.

Ethical consideration is ir.mui.rec. 1394.3.606, the size of samples calculated according to the Cochran formula. That was 120 samples.

Participants aged <50 years and having LGIB in the form of hematochezia or rectorrhagia and with stable hemodynamic were included in the study. Participants with hemodynamic instability, history of colorectal cancer, history of consumption aspirin or anticoagulant, history of previous major abdominal surgery, fair colon preparation, intolerance to free sedation colonoscopy, advance heart and lung disease, documented acute diverticulitis, fulminant colitis, and definitive or suspected perforation were excluded from the study [12]. After cleaning the colon with polyethylene glycol powder with 4–6 l, all colonoscopies were performed without sedation by an experienced gastroenterologist using a Fujinon 4400 Tokyo, Japan Video Scope. If the patients had severe pain and hence used an analgesic, they were excluded. Endoscopic procedures were done in the left lateral position to inhibit aspiration. Details of bowel-cleansing preparation of the colon, initially the patients underwent sigmoidoscopy considered it by getting the scope of colonoscopy from anal canal to splenic flexure by the end of this stage; the levels of the pain and the comfort of the test by physician and patient were measured with visual analog scale from 0 to 10 (10: without discomfort and 0: the most discomfort), duration of procedure were calculated in minutes, and pathologic finding were registered and considered as sigmoidoscopy group. In same patients, the procedure continued until the splenic flexure passed in the ileocecal valve, and this stage was considered as proximal colonoscopy and then from the splenic flexure to ileocecal valve easy performance of this test for the physician and the patient were measured with visual analog scale from zero to ten (10: without discomfort and 0: the most discomfort), duration of procedure to the minute and diagnosed lesions were recorded.

1.1 Statistical analysis

Data were analyzed using IBM SPSS/PC statistical software version 20, the descriptive analysis was based on mean ± standard deviation, and quantitative variable analysis was based on number (%). Compression of comfort for patient and physician and time taken in sigmoidoscopy from splenic flexure to reach ileocecal valve were analyzed by paired *t*-test, and comparisons between the pathologic findings in sigmoidoscopy and full colonoscopy were analyzed by McNemar test.

2. Results

During this study, 120 patients were studied, among which 66 women (55%) and 54 men (45%) participated. The mean of age participants in this study was 41 ± 7.9 years.

According to **Table 1**, and using paired *t*-test, proximal colonoscopy from splenic flexure to reach cecum was relatively easier for the physician and the patient than sigmoidoscopy ($P < 0.001$). Furthermore, the time spent to carry out proximal colonoscopy was less than the time taken for sigmoidoscopy ($P < 0.001$).

In **Table 2**, and using McNemar test, pathologic findings were compared to each other on the basis of doing sigmoidoscopy alone from the anal phase to the splenic flexure or doing a complete colonoscopy from the anus to the cecum. The findings of sigmoidoscopy and the second phase of the procedure (from the splenic flexure to the cecum) have been gathered, and we infer that, based on the table, pathologic findings in full colonoscopy and the findings of sigmoidoscopy showed a significant difference. It means that if the patients underwent full colonoscopy, the pathologic findings show statistically significant differences compared to doing sigmoidoscopy alone.

Variable	Mean±SD		*P*
	Sigmoidoscopy	Splenic flexure till ileocecal	
Feasibility for patient	7.2±1.9	8.2±1.5	>0.001
Feasibility for physician	7±2.3	8.5±1.4	>0.001
Time (min)	6.9±2	3.9±1.4	>0.001

SD=Standard deviation

Table 1.
Compression of feasibility for patient and physician and time in sigmoidoscopy with splenic flexure till ileocecal valve.

Finding	Sigmoidoscopy, *n* (%)	Full colonoscopy, *n* (%)	*P*
Adenoma	10 (9.7)	16 (13.8)	0.014
Cancer	3 (2.8)	4 (3.5)	0.37
Colitis	5 (4.9)	8 (7)	0.04
Angiodysplasia	0	1 (0.9)	0.31
Lipoma	0	1 (0.9)	0.31
Hemorrhoid	70 (67)	70 (60)	1
Diverticula	14 (13.6)	14 (12)	1
Infectious colitis	2 (2)	2 (1.9)	1
Total	104	116	<0.001

Table 2.
The comparison between the pathologic findings in sigmoidoscopy and full colonoscopy.

3. Discussion

The purpose of this study was to investigate the easiness of physician and the patient and the rate of discovering pathologic findings through sigmoidoscopy and full colonoscopy in patients under 50 years old with LGIB. According to the results of this study, doing proximal colonoscopy compared to sigmoidoscopy is easier for the patient and the physician, and the time spent was also less compared to sigmoidoscopy. It seems logical that sigmoidoscopy is more difficult for the patient and physician despite intubation and passing from the rectosigmoid area. According to the pathological findings, it is assumed that the full colonoscopy has been of more diagnostic value for patients because of finding important pathologies. The results were compared with sigmoidoscopy, which indicate a significant difference between the levels of pathological findings in colonoscopy compared to sigmoidoscopy. The pathological findings in colonoscopy were higher than sigmoidoscopy.

LGIB or rectal bleeding is considered as a common concern in the young people, and there is difficulty in making decision about sigmoidoscopy or full colonoscopy. As a whole, it is accepted that full colonoscopy should be performed for the people older than 50 years old with rectal bleeding, but there is no consensus guideline for patients under 50 years yet. In many studies, the researchers have shown that due to this matter, the LGIB or rectal bleeding is considered a common concern in the young people and the benign anorectal pathologies such as hemorrhoids and other concerns are the cause of 90% of rectal bleeding; colorectal cancer increases with age, the method of sigmoidoscopy is sufficient, and there is no need for colonoscopy [11]. However, in several studies including the study performed by Wong et al. [13], 223 patients under 50 years old underwent colonoscopy. Among them, 4 patients (1.8%) had colon cancer in distal colon, 22 patients (9.9%) had adenoma, 6 patients had proximal polyps, and 60.5% of patients had hemorrhoids. They argued that colon cancer can occur in younger persons. Hence, in colonoscopy, it should be strongly considered that the results of this study are consistent with the current study [13], or in the study of Van Rosendaal et al. performed in 2002, from 66 patients, colonoscopy was done in 55 patients, and most of them had the lesion in 60 cm interval of the anus, but there was a cancerous and a polyp lesion upper than 60 cm [14]. In a study by Lewis et al. that was performed to investigate the cause of rectal bleeding in the young people, they concluded that doing colonoscopy in patients between 25 and 45 years is incremental cost-effectiveness [15]. Inconsistent with our study in the study of Aravindan [16], 516 patients were reviewed. They were treated by sigmoidoscopy because of rectal bleeding. Among them, 39 patients (39%) had polyps, and among them 31 cases were rectal, and 8 were sigmoid. Due to their histology, 1.7% was adenomatous, in one patient was rectal carcinoid, and in two patients (0.4%) was carcinoma, and in the other patients, there were hyperplastic polyps. The researchers showed that the prevalence of polyps with large size and advanced adenoma is very low in young people [16], or in another study performed by Khalid et al. [17], they showed that 379 patients who were under 40 years had LGIB and were treated by full colonoscopy. Among them, seven adenomatous polyps and malignant lesions were discovered that all were in the distal colon. In persons at the age of 40–50 years, ten polyps and malignant lesions were discovered that one of them was in the proximal colon. They concluded that most of the lesions were in the distal colon; therefore, flexible sigmoidoscopy is sufficient, and there was no need for full colonoscopy [17]. Furthermore, in another study performed by Nikpour et al. [18], 402 patients with rectal bleeding underwent colonoscopy. Among them, 54.2% had hemorrhoid, 14.2% had anal fissure, and 14.2 had ulcerative colitis which are the most prevalent pathologies. Among 121 patients, 30.1% had significant lesions, 6.5% had adenocarcinoma, and 7.5% had adenomatous polyps, and they finally concluded that the flexible sigmoidoscopy for the patients under 50 years with LGIB can be sufficient [18].

In the current study, there were six pathologic findings beyond splenic flexure (5%) and one cancer beyond splenic flexure (0.8%) and totally 5.8% lesions beyond splenic flexure. These data are significant in young people. Most studies on young people with rectal bleeding recommended sigmoidoscopy for them; one reason is that most of these studies were performed in the west, and in these countries, the colorectal cancer is less common. However, the colorectal cancer in South Asian countries is more complex and is more frequent among young people [19, 20]. It seems reasonable that in these countries such as Iran, the young patients with rectal bleeding should be evaluated by full colonoscopy. On the other hand, in young people, most pathologies causing LGIB are the benign anorectal lesions, but it may be the colorectal lesions need the full colonoscopy. According to our results, most discovered lesions in these patients are anorectal lesions and hemorrhoids that these results are consistent with the other studies as the other observed lesions have been distal colon. According to our results, if in the patients, from the beginning, full colonoscopy was performed, the numbers of discovered pathologies in colonoscopy would be higher than sigmoidoscopy, and it is significantly different ($P < 0.001$). In our study, even though the cost of procedure was increased, the time and comfort of the procedure do not differ from sigmoidoscopy, and the rate of diagnosis of lesions increased; therefore, it is advised that in patients under 50 years and with LGIB, full colonoscopy was considered, especially in Iranian people. Anatomy of the colon was different in Iran from western countries. In Iran, because of high-fiber diet, the sigmoid colon is usually more tortuous and elongated than in western countries. Therefore, sigmoidoscopy is more complicated and time-spending procedure more than expected in western countries. As the result, total colonoscopy is more helpful than sigmoidoscopy as diagnostic procedure and needs less time to do.

Since our sample size is small and there is no personal guideline for doing colonoscopy or sigmoidoscopy in patients under 50 years, and due to ethical issues, we did full colonoscopy for all patients, and we did not have two distinct separate groups to investigate the variables such as age and sex individually in each group. It is recommended that this study be performed in larger sample size and done in two separate groups to use the results in the studies.

4. Conclusions

With regard to this matter, if these patients were under full colonoscopy from the beginning, the satisfaction level in colonoscopy has statistically significant difference with sigmoidoscopy, and it is recommended that the patients under 50 years with rectal bleeding should be under full colonoscopy.

Author details

Mahsa Khodadoostan[1], Ahmad Shavakhi[1], Reihaneh Padidarnia[2]*, Alireza Shavakhi[3] and Mehdi Ahmadian[1]

1 Department of Gastroenterology and Hepatology, Isfahan University of Medical Sciences, Isfahan, Iran

2 Department of Internal Medicine, Isfahan University of Medical Sciences, Isfahan, Iran

3 Shahrekord of Medical University, Shahrekord, Iran

*Address all correspondence to: r.padidarnia@gmail.com

References

[1] Ghassemi KA, Jensen DM. Lower GI bleeding: Epidemiology and management. Current Gastroenterology Reports. 2013;**15**:333

[2] Oakland K, Guy R, Uberoi R, Hogg R, Mortensen N, Murphy MF, et al. Acute lower GI bleeding in the UK: Patient characteristics, interventions and outcomes in the first nationwide audit. Gut. 2017

[3] James R. Management of acute lower gastrointestinal bleeding: Principles and current practice in the United Kingdom. Neoplasia Cancer Polyp. 2015;**17**:8-36

[4] Pasha SF, Shergill A, Acosta RD, Chandrasekhara V, Chathadi KV, et al. The role of endoscopy in the patient with lower GI bleeding. Gastrointestinal Endoscopy. 2014;**79**:875-885

[5] Strate LL. Lower GI bleeding: Epidemiology and diagnosis. Gastroenterology Clinics of North America. 2005;**34**:643-664

[6] Barnert J, Messmann H. Diagnosis and management of lower gastrointestinal bleeding. Nature Reviews. Gastroenterology & Hepatology. 2009;**6**:637-646

[7] Ferguson MA. Office evaluation of rectal bleeding. Clinics in Colon and Rectal Surgery. 2005;**18**:249-254

[8] Korkis AM, McDougall CJ. Rectal bleeding in patients less than 50 years of age. Digestive Diseases and Sciences. 1995;**40**:1520-1523

[9] Strate LL, Syngal S. Predictors of utilization of early colonoscopy vs. radiography for severe lower intestinal bleeding. Gastrointestinal Endoscopy. 2005;**61**:46-52

[10] Angtuaco TL, Reddy SK, Drapkin S, Harrell LE, Howden CW. The utility of urgent colonoscopy in the evaluation of acute lower gastrointestinal tract bleeding: A 2-year experience from a single center. The American Journal of Gastroenterology. 2001;**96**:1782-1785

[11] Lhewa DY, Strate LL. Pros and cons of colonoscopy in management of acute lower gastrointestinal bleeding. World Journal of Gastroenterology. 2012;**18**:1185-1190

[12] Zuccar G Jr. Management of the adult patient with acute lower gastrointestinal bleeding. American College of Gastroenterology. 1998;**93**:1202-1218

[13] Wong RF, Khosla R, Moore JH, Kuwada SK. Consider colonoscopy for young patients with hematochezia. The Journal of Family Practice. 2004;**53**:879-884

[14] Van Rosendaal GM, Sutherland LR, Verhoef MJ, Bailey RJ, Blustein PK, Lalor EA, et al. Defining the role of fiberoptic sigmoidoscopy in the investigation of patients presenting with bright red rectal bleeding. The American Journal of Gastroenterology. 2000;**95**:1184-1187

[15] Lewis JD, Brown A, Localio AR, Schwartz JS. Initial evaluation of rectal bleeding in young persons: A cost-effectiveness analysis. Annals of Internal Medicine. 2002;**136**:99-110

[16] Aravindan N. The value of flexible sigmoidoscopy in the evaluation of rectal bleeding in the young. International Journal of Surgery. 2016;**2**:214-217

[17] Khalid AB, Majid S, Salih M, Hashmat F, Jafri W. Is full colonoscopic examination necessary in young patients with fresh bleeding per rectum? Endoscopy. 2011;**43**:692-696

[18] Nikpour S, Ali Asgari A. Colonoscopic evaluation of minimal rectal bleeding in average-risk patients for colorectal cancer. World Journal of Gastroenterology. 2008;**14**:6536-6540

[19] Deo SV, Shukla NK, Srinivas G, Mohanti BK, Raina V, Sharma A, et al. Colorectal cancers—Experience at a regional cancer centre in India. Tropical Gastroenterology. 2001;**22**:83-86

[20] Shaikh AJ, Raza S, Shaikh AA, Idress R, Kumar S, Rasheed YA, et al. Demographics, pathologic patterns and long-term survival in operable colon cancers: Local experience in Pakistan. Asian Pacific Journal of Cancer Prevention. 2009;**10**:361-364

Chapter 6

Radioimaging Diagnosis of Vaterian Ampulloma: Technique, Semiology, and Differential Diagnosis - Review

Ana Magdalena Bratu and Constantin Zaharia

Abstract

The lining of the Vater papilla represents a complex set of folds of the mucous membrane which acts as an anti-reflux valve and participates in regulating the flow in pancreatic and biliary secretion. The constitutive smooth muscles of the Oddi sphincter differ both anatomically and especially embryologically from the parietal duodenal muscles. This is one of the reasons why some authors believe that the vaterian ampulloma is a distinct oncologic entity from the rest of the duodenal or pancreatic primitive neoplasia. The variations of the implantation manner in the papilla of the common bile duct and pancreatic one simultaneously determine different ways of surgical approach of malignancies of this region. Radioimaging diagnostic methods in suspected vaterian ampulloma require a more special technique. The purpose of this paper is to determine the potential semiological, radiological, and imaging characteristics that will allow a diagnosis of vaterian ampulloma, considering that the surgical therapy, as well as the survival rate in patients, is different from the other neoplasm of the region.

Keywords: vaterian ampulloma, duodenum, barium meal, duodenography, computed tomography, MRI, vaterian ampulloma

1. Introduction

The region of the ampulla of Vater is an anatomical and functional complex, a separate entity, mainly comprising the biliopancreaticoduodenal confluence area. The ampulla territory includes in its structure the terminal portion of the choledoch, including the Oddi sphincter and the main duct of Wirsung, forming the papilla at the duodenal level. In 85% of cases, the openings of the main bile duct and the pancreatic canal are common. The terminal choledoch, after crossing the duodenal wall, next to the duct of Wirsung, opens in the ampulla of Vater. The choledoch implants in the papilla is variable. In most cases, the choledoch has a tangential implantation through the duodenal wall, reaching the level of the ampulla, the choledoch ends differently, either with a highly developed sphincter in the case of a small ampulla or with a much less developed sphincter in the case of a well-highlighted ampulla [1].

The localization of the papilla at the duodenum level is in most cases on the medial contour of the descending duodenum, at the junction of the middle third with the lower third, but ectopic positions of the papilla are known, cranial at 1–2 cm below the bulb level, or caudal at the lower duodenal knee level [1].

A special place is occupied by the cancers of the ampulla of Vater, which are distinct entities, separate from those of the duodenum, although the anatomical location of the ampulla of Vater is at the level of the descending duodenum, due to their embryological origins and the different histological structures [1].

Neoplasms of the vaterian region, also known as vaterian ampulloma, may have as a starting point the cylindrical choledochal epithelium, the Wirsungian cubic epithelium, or the glandular epithelium of the papilla. Due to their origin in an epithelial type tissue structure, histopathologically these tumors are adenocarcinomas [1].

2. Radioimaging techniques of the duodenopancreatic region

The involvement of the duodenum in the neighboring tumor pathology is explained primarily by the multitude of anatomical direct relationships that this organ has with the pancreas, liver, right kidney, colonic hepatic angle, etc.

Neoplasms of the vicinity that have been shown to be invasive in the duodenum are pancreatic tumors, regardless of the segment of this organ, hepatomas, gallbladder cancers, cholangiocarcinomas, malignancies of the right kidney, and colonic, retroperitoneal, as well as gastric duodenal lymphoma. Of these, the most common are the pancreatic neoplasms and the vaterian ampullomas [1].

From our experience, duodenal neoplasms can reach 13% of the total number of neoplasms of the pancreatic-duodenal region, most common being the invasive pancreatic cancer in the duodenum, with a percentage reaching up to 65%, followed by the vaterian ampullomas with a frequency of over 10% [1].

Talamini et al. [2] considers in a study conducted over a 28-year period that ampullary adenocarcinomas are the second most common malignancy in the periampullary region. In the present work, the vaterian ampullomas are in second place by frequency, after the pancreatic neoplasms, but in a ratio equal to the duodenal malignancies themselves.

The objectives of the radio-imagistic explorations in the vaterian ampulloma are:

- Detection of the tumor lesion, providing information on the location, shape, dimensions, and contours of the space replacement process, as well as on the presence of any ulcerations or fistulas and the degree of lumen stenosis
- The state of the duodenal mucosa, insisting on the morphofunctional and autoplastic changes
- Modifications of the duodenal papilla
- Changes in size of the duodenal wall
- Extension of the ampullary lesion in the periduodenal space
- The existence of modifications of the parenchymatous organs or segments of the digestive tract potentially involved in the mechanisms of tumor onset or the degree of tumor invasion in the neighboring organs
- The existence of possible subdiaphragmatic adenopathies

2.1 Radiological exploration

2.1.1 Conventional radiological examination: barium meal

By its anatomical location, any lesion at the level of the ampulla of Vater requires the radiological study of the duodenal framework, especially the descending duodenum.

Examination of the duodenum follows that of the stomach, which is why some aspects are difficult to highlight or elude the examiner due to technical defects or because he is distracted by the presence of other concomitant or associated lesions of the esophagus or stomach.

2.1.1.1 Simple contrast technique

The technique of examining the duodenum using simple contrast is that used in routine examination, following that of the esophagus and the stomach [1]. During this examination the patient ingests 240–360 ml of barium sulfate suspension in water, concentration 30–40%. It is preferable for the contrast agent to have small particles with a high dispersion degree of 4000–6000 particles/cm^2. For a better adhesion of the contrast agent to the mucosal folds, it is recommended to associate a homogenizing agent such as methyl cellulose in the barium sulfate suspension.

Preparation of the patient in the event of a suspected vaterian ampulloma should be done with great care, including an adequate diet, avoiding fermentable foods, long-molecule cellulose, and excess lipids, prohibiting any food intake 6–8 hours before examination, or secretion evacuation if the existence of a stenosis is a certainty. In order not to modify the functional duodenal mechano-secretory behavior, it is advisable to avoid the administration of drugs with implication in the duodenopancreatic physiology.

In this method of examination, the bulb and the rest of the duodenal frame are filled with contrast agent due to gravity and normal peristaltic movements of the stomach, the patient being in orthostatism, ventral decubitus, or right lateral decubitus.

The technique of simple contrast duodenal exploration is a routine examination. It can be performed at any radiology office. However, the method also has drawbacks, the main ones being the overlap of the antrum and the sometimes-insufficient distension of the duodenum.

2.1.1.2 Double-contrast technique

This technique can be mainly achieved in two ways [1]:

a. Double-contrast hypotonic duodenography

b. Probe duodenography

2.1.1.2.1 Double-contrast hypotonic duodenography

Evaluation of the duodenum in double contrast may be part of the standard double contrast of the upper gastrointestinal tract. The examination starts with the carrying out of a seriography after ingesting a single barium swallow that allows a good lining of the digestive mucosa; this represents the mucographic time. At the same time, the exact position of the different portions of the gastric segment is noted.

The double-contrast hypotonic duodenography can be obtained using two methods: the double-contrast method performed during the eso-gastro-duodenal examination, using glucagon and a gaseous potion as a pharmacodynamics, or the hypotonic duodenography in which the patient is given an antispastic after administration of the contrast agent.

In the first method, the double-contrast phase can be obtained by inducing a short-term hypotonia by injecting 0.1 mg of glucagon IV at the beginning of the examination, after which the patient ingests the gaseous agent, respectively, a mixture of citric acid and sodium bicarbonate, with 10 ml of water and high-density barium sulfate, of about 200–250 wt/vol%. After 5–10 min, during which the esophagus and stomach are examined, the hypotonic effect of the glucagon is finished so that the air and barium pass easily through the pylorus and reach the duodenum. The positioning of the patient in ventral and left posterior oblique decubitus fills the duodenal bulb with high-density barium. The compression performed in ventral decubitus is not as useful as in simple contrast due to the increased barium density. We can obtain a series of double-contrast images of both the bulb and duodenal frame in the right anterior oblique position after the patient ingests 240 ml of low-density barium suspension.

The method has maximum reliability for examining the stomach, duodenal bulb, and possibly the descending duodenum. It has the disadvantage that it does not allow a good assessment of the state of the duodenal mucosa, and the overlaps of the antral portion cannot always be excluded. Also, the two fractions of barium suspension can be mixed, which may induce interpretation errors.

In the second method, the exploration is required to be carried out quickly; the patient should swallow 100–150 ml of barium sulfate suspension. The patient is placed in dorsal decubitus, then the antispastic is injected, after which the subject is immediately repositioned in the right lateral decubitus, a position in which he ingests the effervescent potion through a pipette or cannula. The contrast agent enters the duodenum which is already in hypotonic state. The duodenum in repletion and hypotonia is radiographed in this position and in several incidences in left posterior oblique position. The duodenal distension fades in dorsal decubitus and the root of the mesentery no longer ensuring its compression on D3. An accumulation of contrast agents is observed in the bulb. In this situation it is sufficient to raise the table by 30° in order to evacuate it and to be able to carry out the correct seriographies on the duodenum, especially the descending portion and the bulb, which, due to the hypotony, expands with the gas released by the effervescent potion.

There is also a method that can prevent overlapping of the gastric antral. This consists of introducing an Einhorn probe into the duodenum and through it 10 ml of xylin, with high viscosity administered at body temperature, which can achieve a hypotonia of the duodenum after a few minutes. Instead of xylin, scobutil can be used, administered intravenously. The hypotonic effect occurs in about 15–30 min. Barium sulfate suspension administration on the probe allows the duodenal framework to be completely opacified.

The method also has disadvantages. Antispasmodics alter the kinetics, tonicity, and duodenal secretion. During this time, due to the induced changes, the duodenal stasis is accentuated. For this reason, the low-density barium sulfate suspension is mixed with the stasis liquid, and if we do not use a homogenizing agent, bubbles may appear at the air-liquid interface that can fix themselves on the mucous folds, leading to an erroneous diagnosis. The method gives exclusively morphological information which means an incomplete radiological diagnosis. Due to hypotonia and hypokinesia, any stiffness and the study of autoplasty cannot be properly appreciated.

2.1.1.2.2 Selective duodenography or probe duodenography

This method is used when the radiologist is interested in studying the duodenal framework or when, following previous examinations, the suspicion of a strictly localized lesion at this level is raised.

An enteral probe is used to perform this technique. The probe is introduced nasally or orally after the pharyngeal mucosa is embrocated or anesthetic solution is gargled. The distal end of the probe should reach the mid-level of D2; insertion of the probe into the stomach is done with the patient in a seated position, after which the patient lies in a right lateral decubitus and the probe is passed through the pylorus. To avoid coiling the probe, it is good to use either a probe weighted at the end or a metallic, soft, and flexible guide. The positioning of the probe will be done under radioscopic control. Then the duodenum is aspirated, after which the barium suspension is introduced under pressure, in a volume of about 30–50 ml. The suspension of barium sulfate must be fluid, homogeneous, and very adherent. It is indicated that the barium sulfate has a high dispersion degree and the suspension contains a methyl cellulose-type surfactant. Double contrast is obtained by blowing about 80–100 cm^3 of air into the duodenum. The insufflation is gradual, under radioscopic control during examination.

The examination is performed in several positions and incidences, being mandatory to start from dorsal and right oblique anterior decubitus, continuing with the ventral and oblique posterior left decubitus, performing serial X-rays. Highlighting any anomalies requires X-rays of different incidences and intermediate positions, being able to better highlight the lesion.

The results are good, but they require a perfect knowledge of the anatomy of the region and the normal radiological aspect, since it differs from the known radiological anatomy.

The main advantage of the method is that it is possible to avoid overlaps with other segments of the digestive tract, especially with the gastric antrum. Also, by this method, small lesions of the mucosa can be detected, which can elude the examiner in simple contrast or in double contrast performed during the eso-gastro-duodenal examination. Antispastic substances that modify normal duodenal tonicity and kinetics and which modify duodenal secretion are not used. In this way the examination can also provide functional data of the investigated segment.

The examination is unpleasant for the patient due to the need to introduce the probe; therefore it is advisable that the examination be preceded by a brief discussion with the subject, in which the technique and the need for the examination will be explained to him. The crossing of the pylorus cannot always be realized; at position changes, a withdrawal of the probe into the stomach can occur, an incident that can also occur at a sharp intake of breath. This can be avoided if the examination is performed using a probe with a balloon at the end, which will set it to the desired level. The advantage of using such a probe is to prevent airflow back into the gastric antrum.

The time required for the examination is long. The technique is not of first intention, usually being performed only when there are clear clinical indications about the presence of a space replacement process.

The radiological techniques described can assess the overall duodenal morphology. Under distension and hypotony, the duodenal frame as a whole appears slightly enlarged. The examination allows to identify the duodenal anatomical segments and their possible anatomical variants (reverse V duodenum, mobile duodenum, small duodenal frame, surrounding the bulb, as in the case of gastric ptosis).

On the postero-external border of the descending duodenum, it is possible to highlight a possible imprint, due to the direct relations with the right kidney at this level.

Duodenal distension is exercised up to the level of its horizontal portion, immediately after the lower knee, when the examination is performed in ventral and oblique posterior left decubitus, being determined by the compression of the mesenter's root over D3; in dorsal decubitus the compression is attenuated.

In dorsal decubitus the large papilla is visualized as a round-oval or oval transparency, contoured by the contrast substance. This area corresponds to the intramural pathway of the choledoch. The surrounding, well-visualized folds can converge into a single longitudinal fold or a bifid fold. The small papilla is rarely seen as a round lacunar image, with a diameter of about 5 mm, located cranially and medially to the large papilla.

In lateral decubitus, the longitudinal fold is highlighted on the endoluminal face, and the external duodenal contour becomes rectilinear due to the distension that erases the connivent valves. At the place of formation of the longitudinal fold, toward the tuber, a notch can be distinguished, which corresponds to the choledochian sphincter at this level. The small papilla is sometimes viewed as a notch located cranially to the large papilla.

Conventional radiological techniques represent at this time methods that are really historical, computed tomography replacing almost all of them.

2.1.2 Computed tomography

Technological progress (much shorter scanning time, better spatial resolution) and the new adapted examination protocols allow accurate study of the digestive wall and extra-parietal lesion extension [1, 3–8].

The main problem is obtaining an optimal distension of the duodenum in order to be able to correctly estimate the thickness of its wall, which is the most important computed tomography criterion of normality.

The duodenum is the most difficult region to examine due to the difficulty of obtaining adequate opacity, this being determined by the accelerated transport of water into the lumen, the water that dilutes the contrast agent.

Therefore, for the study of the duodenum, in fact of the entire upper digestive floor, the CT scan must be preceded by the ingestion of 600 ml of iodinated, water-soluble contrast substance, in a dilution of 2–3% approx. 5–10 min beforehand. IV antispastics can also be associated, which allow for a good study of the duodenal framework and the dissociation of the pancreas head. The exclusive use of air distension, as well as the use of simple water in combination with gastroduodenal hypotonia, increases the quality of parietography. The normal thickness of the duodenal wall is considered to be 3–4 mm.

The use of antispasmodics administered IV may diminish the artifacts generated by peristalsis, but due to the current ability to use a scanning time of less than 5 seconds, it is no longer of interest.

The intravenous administration of the iodinated contrast agent should be systematic for assessing the iodophilia of the lesion and for studying the relationships with the neighboring structures. It is also used to assess the extent of the tumor lesion, by determining the metastases, as well as to assess the existence of any abnormalities in the parenchymal organs, in relation to the duodenal disease or simultaneous with it.

In view of the frequent involvement of the duodenum in the neighboring tumors, especially those in the pancreas, in the vaterian ampulloma, etc., performing the computed tomographic examination both native and with contrast agent becomes almost obligatory. Thus, computed tomography becomes the essential method of establishing the starting point in duodenal tumor determinations, at the same time achieving the pre-therapeutic balance of the lesion extension.

The administration of the intravenous contrast substance allows at the same time to opacify the vascular landmarks of this region, particularly the renal vein, inferior vena cava, as well as of the superior splenic and mesenteric vessels. The possibility of conducting the spiral computed tomographic examination gives almost overlapping information with the angiographic examination.

The acquisition is made through contiguous sections, 5 mm thick, but 3 mm sections can be used to allow analysis of small organs or to obtain details on the lesion.

The patient is initially placed in dorsal decubitus. The computed tomographic examination can be complemented, depending on the needs, with sections performed in ventral decubitus, lateral decubitus, sections that highlight the digestive connection of large tumor masses, and their dissociation from the adjacent viscera.

The use of some image processing techniques allows biplane or spatial reconstruction of the bile ducts and the duct of Wirsung and is usually used to detect lesions of distal bile ducts and in the vaterian ampulloma.

2.2 Imaging explorations

2.2.1 Ultrasound

Ultrasonography as an imaging exploration of the duodenum is not a primary intention technique [1, 9]. It can be performed transabdominally—routine examination in which the primary information is related to the pathology of the parenchymal organs—and echoendoscopy, a method with maximum reliability on the pathology of the duodenal wall and the eventual differential diagnosis between primitive duodenal lesions/invasion by contiguity.

If the first technique of ultrasonographic exploration has a general addressability and accessibility, not requiring a special training of the patient, the second technique requires special equipment and a special skillset, being used especially by the doctors performing endoscopy, as a complement to a routine endoscopic examination.

Transparietal ultrasound can reveal changes of the duodenal peristaltic, duodenal stasis, or parietal duodenal infiltration. Complementing the examination with the Doppler technique may bring additional information to the duodenal tumor pathology. Probes of at least 5 MHz should be used for better lesion detection.

Ultrasound examination of the pancreas and distal bile ducts is the primary method for any suspected tumor pathology.

The specificity and sensitivity of the method depend on the quality of the equipment, but in particular, on the experience of the one using the method.

2.2.2 MRI

MRI scanning is not a primary imaging technique for patients with suspected tumor pathology of the duodenum-pancreatic region [1, 10–17]. The possibility of clearly highlighting soft structures and multiplane images makes this method superior to computer tomographic exploration. Magnetic resonance highlights both the duodenal wall and the intraluminal duodenal content.

The body antenna is most commonly used. The spin echo sequences are constituted as reference sequences. T1-weighted sequences with short TR and TE allow excellent spatial resolution, providing the best morphological information of abdominal viscera.

T2-weighted sequences with long TR and TE have a good resolution in contrast and allow a more reliable tissue study. Given the relatively long acquisition time, at least 3 min, FLASH or SPGR gradient echo sequences are used more frequently, although they have a lower signal-to-noise ratio.

The use of fat saturation sequences reduces respiratory and structural artifacts but has a longer acquisition time.

For a complete study, it is absolutely necessary to use sequences specific to the study of vessels.

In case of suspicion of an ampullary tumor, MRCP is mandatory. In the last three decades, this technique has become absolutely necessary in the diagnosis of a biliary duct obstruction, obstruction which is caused at the right level by an ampullary tumor. MRCP is a diagnostic method, while ERCP remained a rather interventional method. T2 hyperintensive sequences are used, which make the content of both biliary and Wirsung ducts white in contrast to the rest of the structures. Sequences with thin sections (3–5 mm), which have the purpose of an MIP type reconstruction, and sequences with thick sections (30–50 mm), which have a short acquisition time (<5 s) and which are performed in multiple planes, are used. The acquisitions are made in the coronal and oblique coronal plane. If we refer strictly to MRCP, the administration of the contrast agent is not obligatory, but in the case of the ampullary tumors, this is a complementary sequence that is associated with the abdominal MRI scan. The MRCP highlights the contents and implicitly the size of the bile ducts and the duct of Wirsung, but does not give details on their wall, which was done by an abdominal MRI scan.

However, with MRCP you can administer negative oral contrast agent that reduces the hypersignal of gastric and intestinal fluids, thus increasing the contrast of the contents of the bile ducts and the duct of Wirsung.

In addition, the MRCP technique can provide information on the pancreatic function. This is achieved by the intravenous administration of secretin which has the role of increasing the pancreatic exocrine function, so it will increase the flow and quantity of pancreatic juice, and implicitly it will expand to the maximum the pancreatic ducts, thus being able to highlight both the main duct and the secondary ones.

The axial plane examination constitutes the reference sequences of the examination. In order to specify the exact anatomical reports or for the study of the vessels, frontal and coronal acquisitions are also made.

The mucosal study is performed using water per os or more reliably through the probe. The study of parietal changes requires sequences with paramagnetic contrast products.

The MR exploration, due to the possibilities of acquisition, processing, and reconstruction of the images, allows the study of the biliary ducts, having major importance in the tumor pathology of the duodenopancreatic region and the study dedicated to the vessels related to this region.

3. Semiology of ampulla of Vater neoplasms

The histological structure comprises the tunics of the duodenal wall but also a separate muscular entity—the Oddi sphincter [1]. In terms of structure, the smooth musculature of the Oddi sphincter differs both anatomically and embryologically from the surrounding duodenal musculature. Its mechanical and electrical activity is independent and different from that of the duodenal muscle, but it is integrated into myogenic, regulating mechanisms through innervation and hormonal activity.

The mucus of the Vater papilla forms a complicated system of folds whose main function is the creation of "valves" with anti-reflux role, especially for biliary drainage. The ampulla of Vater is visible during the radiological examination in double contrast of the duodenum, being recognizable due to the presence of a superior fold and the longitudinal fold, located on the posteromedial face of the descending duodenum. Frequently at this level, there are two oblique folds. In conventional radiological exploration, in simple contrast, visualization of the papilla is much more difficult.

These are briefly some of the anatomical, functional, and embryological arguments that cause the tumor pathology of the ampulla of Vater to be treated separately from that of the duodenum, although the location of the Vater papilla is at the level of the descending duodenum, approximately in the middle of it.

These considerations have a very important practical substrate. According to Dudiak et al. [7], there is a direct interrelation between the anatomy and the embryology of the papilla and the radiological and endoscopic exploration possibilities, but especially in interventional radiology and endoscopy.

3.1 Radioimaging changes found in ampulla of Vater neoplasms

Regardless of the radioimaging method used, in the case of neoplasms of the ampulla of Vater, several signs that can guide the diagnosis can be highlighted (**Figure 1**).

Computed tomography and magnetic resonance imaging are particularly reliable in diagnosing cancers of the ampulla of Vater (**Figures 2** and **3**).

Next we tried an analysis of these signs, direct or indirect, which alone or associated would help the radiologist to diagnose the lesion as accurately as possible.

3.2 The lacuna

The classical radiological appearance of the ampullar neoplasm consists of a lacunar image located in the region of the ampulla of Vater, which can be located intraluminally or marginally, on the internal contour of the second portion of the duodenum. This radiological change is also mentioned as a radiological sign of probability of a vaterian ampulloma by Caroli et al. [18].

The lacuna, as an elementary change in the radiological diagnosis of the ampulla, has lost its importance with the advent of other techniques of radioimaging investigation. In view of its existence, relatively frequently encountered today in standard radiological exploration protocols, we introduced the analysis of this radiological sign in this study as well.

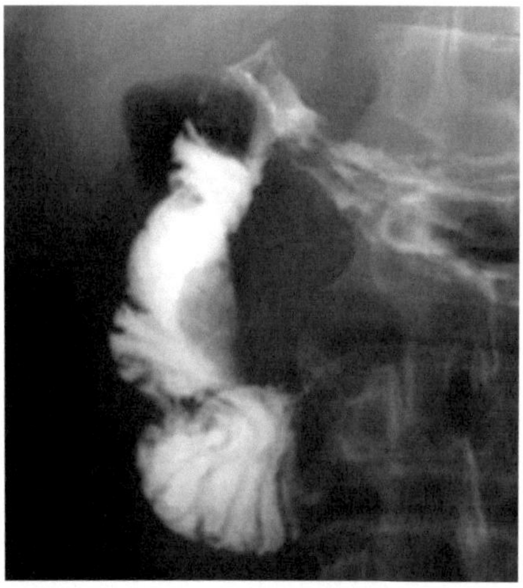

Figure 1.
Vaterian ampulloma: Conventional exploration.

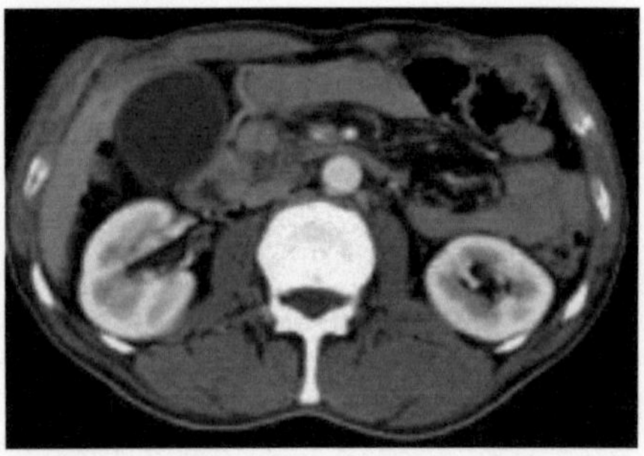

Figure 2.
Vaterian ampulloma: CT exploration.

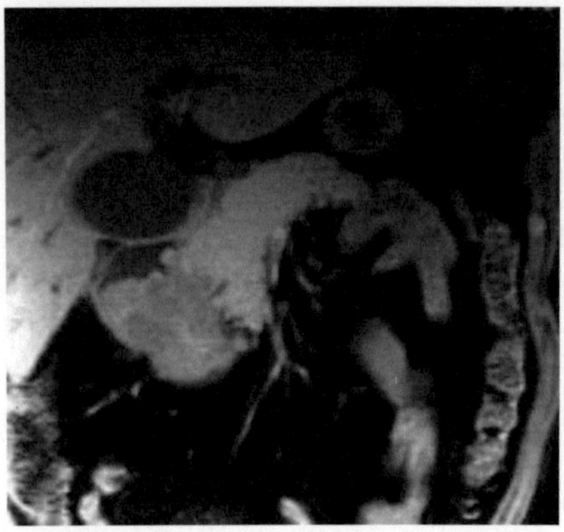

Figure 3.
Vaterian ampulloma: MRI exploration.

The lacuna can be highlighted in a percentage of less than 40% of the total cases of malignancies of the pancreatic-duodenal region [1] (**Figure 4**).

The standardized criteria of malignancy of a lacuna considers that it must have an irregular and erased contour; it must interrupt the folds, due to peritumoral malignant infiltration, coexisting with the presence of possible superficial ulcerations; and, in principle, it is larger than 2–3 cm. Although it is known that ampullary carcinomas do not reach overly large sizes until the moment of diagnosis, due to the relatively rapid installation of jaundice, the specialized literature attests the presence of areas of neoplastic cells in the structure of a vaterian adenoma, even of very small dimensions.

Because of this, but also due to the fact that a conventional radiological examination, no matter how well performed, cannot accomplish the benign-malignant differentiation in the case of ampullary tumors, we consider that only the contours and dimensions of the ampullae should be analyzed.

From a dimensional point of view, we classified the lacunas in the ampulloma in gaps with diameters between 1–3, 3–5, and over 5 cm.

It is proven that this neoplastic entity is in the form of a small space replacement process, below 3 cm in a percentage of 70%, the remaining 30% being tumors with dimensions between 3 and 5 cm. You can also see the absence of space replacement processes with dimensions over 5 cm.

Semelka et al. [19], following a study carried out over a 2-year period, regarding the ampullary carcinoma, have concluded that the dimensions of this type of neoplasia do not exceed 5.5 cm.

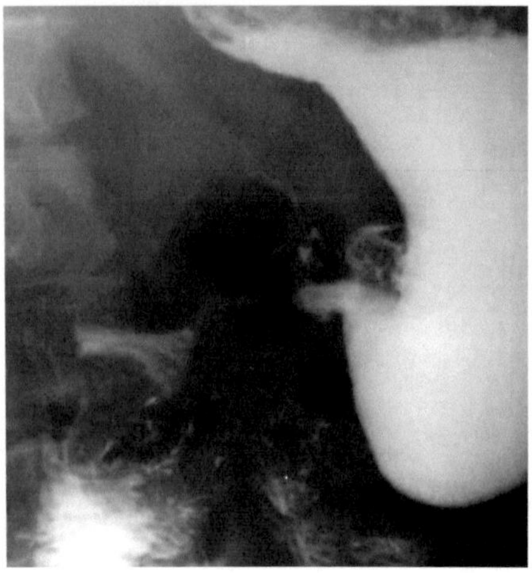

Figure 4.
The lacuna in a vaterian ampulloma.

These are arguments in favor of the authors' assertions that vaterian carcinoma is largely the result of malignant transformation of an adenoma.

Also, the reduced size and the histopathological nature of the ampullary adenocarcinoma lead to the conclusion that this **type** of neoplasm is one with reduced aggressiveness.

The conventional radiological examination is excellently complemented by the computed tomographic exploration or by magnetic resonance that can detect space replacement processes with dimensions up to 1 cm. These are seen as small occurrences in the duodenal lumen, which cannot be detected by the standard radiological examination.

The report of detection of space replacement processes by the two associated methods, the examination of the duodenum in double-contrast and computed tomography or MRI, actually highlights a double number of processes of space replacement at the level of the ampulla of Vater, regardless of its size. Comparison of these two exploration techniques with each other, but also with endoscopic exploration, reveals a greater specificity of magnetic resonance exploration than computed tomographic exploration.

Semelka et al. [19], in a study on the reliability of radiological and imaging scanning techniques versus ERCP, concluded on the superior specificity of magnetic resonance scanning compared to computed tomography. At the same time, considering the potential risks of retrograde endoscopic cholangiopancreatography, it recommends MRI as the diagnostic method with the highest degree of specificity.

In conclusion, we have considered all the radio-imagistic methods of detecting the process of space replacement in the case of the vaterian ampullomas, which we presented at the beginning of this subchapter.

3.3 The presence of the Frostberg sign

The Frostberg sign, also known as the inverted "3" sign (**Figure 5**), represents, from a radiological point of view, a semiological contour modification, which translates into an enlargement of the duodenal papilla, in the center of which the insertion of the biliary and pancreatic ducts remains fixed.

From the etiological point of view, this radiological modification is nonspecific; it can be present both in the malignant tumors of the ampulla of Vater and in any enlargement of the head of the pancreas, whatever the cause.

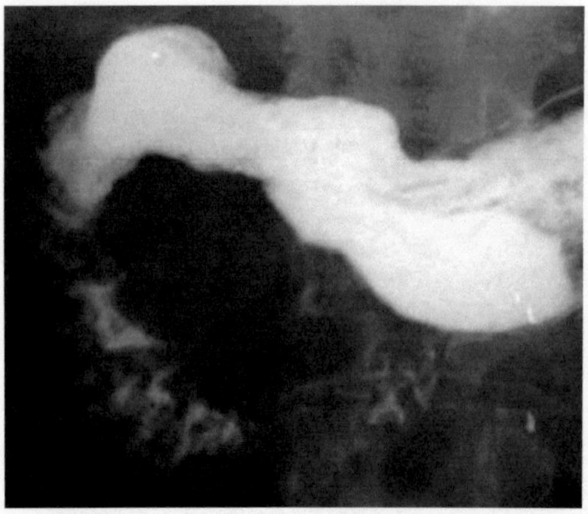

Figure 5.
Frostberg sign.

The existence of Frostberg's sign actually pleads for the secondary invasion of the ampullar "carrefour."

Radiologically the two convexities connected between them represent in fact the edges of the papilla, and the opacified spines between them correspond to filling the papillary orifice with contrast agent.

The existence of the Oddi sphincter, but at the same time the tumor infiltration, does not allow the reflux of the contrast agent neither in the duct of Wirsung nor in the main biliary duct.

The conventional treatises of conventional radiology place Frostberg's sign as the second in frequency in the radiological semiology of the vaterian ampulloma. At the same time, the specificity of this radiological manifestation is relatively small, recognizing that translating the enlargement of the papilla, in fact a papillary suffering, is incriminated, without being able to indicate its substrate.

Ferruci [20] considers the Frostberg sign to be a relatively rare sign, which has specificity with regard to the damage of the duodenal papilla, without being able to define the cause of this change.

The presence of the Frostberg sign in almost 60% of cases is detected in the vaterian ampullomas.

Although not pathognomonic, it is also found in pancreatic disorders; the Frostberg sign is frequently detected in ampullary carcinomas. With it we can differentiate, using the conventional radiological exploration only as a method of investigation, the vaterian ampulloma from the primitive duodenal malignancies. This assertion is based on the fact that any primitive malignant tumor, in which the developing area also includes the papilla, infiltrates the ampullae by erasing its outlines and damaging the specific architecture of the papillary folds.

Being a radiological contour modification, in the case of the double-contrast duodenum examinations, an exploration that achieves the maximum luminal distension is much better highlighted and thus reveals the finest modification of the duodenal contour.

3.4 Rigidity

In the case of ampullary adenocarcinomas, the segmental rigidity, from the level of the internal contour of the descending duodenum, above and/or underlying the tumor lesion, translates the neoplastic invasion by contiguity of the duodenal wall itself.

It is considered that the presence of rigidity on the internal contour of the descending duodenum is a radiological sign, which, associated with the lacuna, gives the radiological image a certain specificity regarding the vaterian ampulloma.

Taking into account the pathophysiological substrate of rigidity and considering that the vaterian ampullomas are neoplasms with reduced aggression, a small percentage of only 20% is explained, so the duodenal invasion is present in less than a quarter of cases [1].

The presence of rigidity is considered important because it is one of the first signs that can be highlighted by the standard radiological examination, especially by the double-contrast probe duodenography, the method that achieves the most reliable distension of the duodenal lumen. Highlighting a segment that presents rigidity, including the duodenal papilla, may be useful in associating the Frostberg sign. In this case, a radiological differential diagnosis can be made between the vaterian ampulloma and papillary disorders of other etiologies. The presence of rigidity in the absence of the Frostberg sign reduces the probability of the existence of a vaterian ampulloma, but it cannot completely exclude this diagnostic possibility. At the opposite pole is the hypotonic duodenography, which, due to the lack of duodenal functional information, highlights the rigidity with more difficulty.

From a dimensional point of view, the rigidity in the case it exists within the vaterian ampulloma has dimensions between 3 and 5 cm.

3.5 The imprint

Ferruci [20] considers the imprint an important sign of conventional radiological exploration in detecting a space replacement process located in the vicinity of the duodenum, without necessarily having the meaning of a neoplasm.

Although it is an intrinsic neoplastic process, the vaterian ampulloma may induce imprinting due to the accompanying pancreatic reaction or, another explanation would be that the vaterian ampulloma invaded the pancreas. Regardless of the nature of the cause in the situation of the vaterian adenocarcinoma, the impression is the result of the dimensional increase at the level of the head of the pancreas.

In the case of the vaterian ampullomas, the imprint is found in up to 20% of cases.

The vaterian neoplasm is not a type of malignancy of the duodenum, but is localized within the duodenum, the vaterian ampulla being not a neighboring organ.

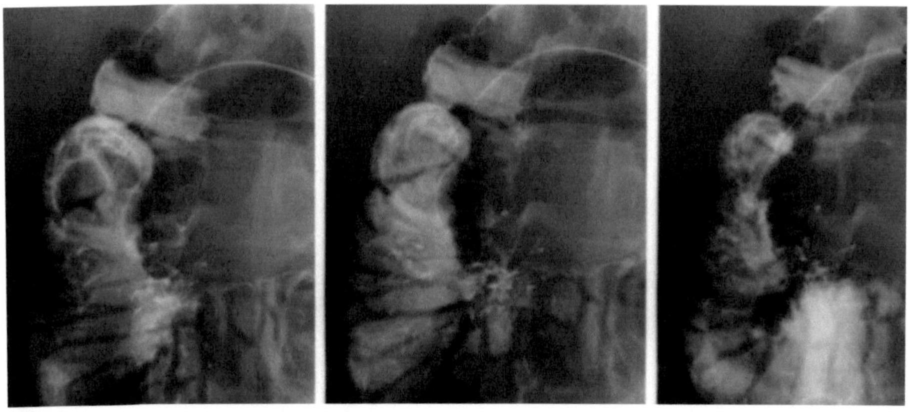

Figure 6.
Vaterian ampulloma: Imprint.

The imprint may occur due to the segmental enlargement of the head of the pancreas, due to the perilesional edema.

In any case, the imprint due to vaterian ampulloma is less spread on the contour of the descending duodenum than in the case of pancreatic cephalic malignancies. In the case of neoplasms with localization in the head of the pancreas, the association of changes in the extremity of the mucosal folds in the vicinity of the neoplasm is mentioned almost constantly, by the appearance of what bears the name of "T fold." Vaterian ampullomas never associate this change in orientation of the mucosal folds (**Figure 6**).

The presence of the imprint could possibly be a radiological sign of differentiation between the duodenal malignancies and the vaterian ampullomas but with a higher specificity between the duodenal tumors and any other tumor spread to the level of the descending duodenum.

3.6 Changes of mucosal folds

Although the tumor process originates from the epithelium of the structures of the ampulla of Vater, its location makes the effect on the duodenal mucosal folds important.

In 70% of vaterian ampullomas, modifications of the mucosal folds are described, and unlike the primitive duodenal malignancies, there are also 30% of cases in which there is no evidence of duodenal mucosal damage.

Alignment of the extremities of the folds on the internal contour of the descending duodenum may indicate a neoplastic process, either ampullary or neighboring—head of the pancreas–but may also be encountered in the case of pancreatitis or perivisceritis, being a nonspecific sign. In the case of the vaterian ampullomas, the alignment of the folds takes place above the papilla (**Figure 7**).

The presence of disorganized folds, although reduced in number, is important from a diagnostic point of view [1], being considered the disorganized folds in the descending duodenum as a sign of damage to the duodenal papilla. It can be concluded that this type of radiological modification cannot differentiate between ampullary malignancies and invasion of the ampulla of Vater by pancreatic cephalic neoplasms.

A more important extension at the level of the duodenal mucosa determines the presence of folds interrupted at the level of the second topographic segment of the duodenum.

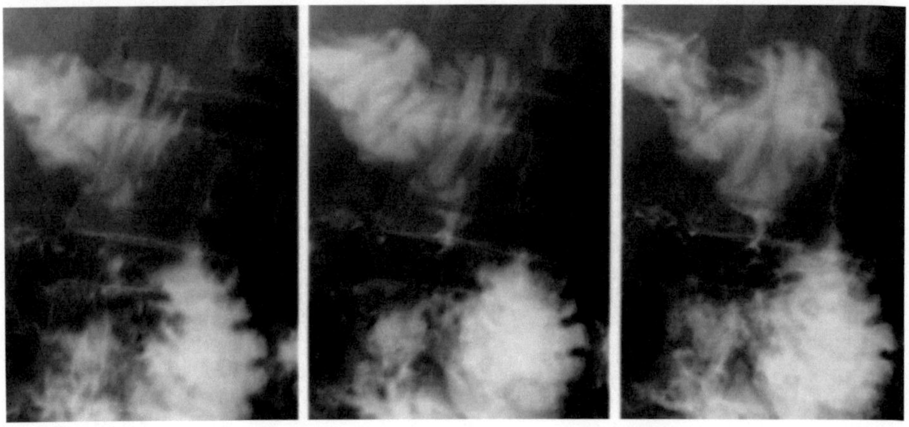

Figure 7.
Folds aligned above the lesion.

The existence of ampulla of Vater adenocarcinoma does not, however, require the disappearance of all mucosal folds at the papilla level. A neoplastic infiltration of the papilla can lead to the deletion of the longitudinal fold and at the same time to a thickening of the superior fold, in which the diagnosis can only be made endoscopically, possibly with the association of multiple biopsies.

It should be noted that the dual contrast method of duodenography allows for a much more reliable study of mucosal folds, especially those at the duodenal papilla level, which requires maximum distension of the duodenal lumen, as well as double-contrast air-barium exploration.

3.7 Thickness of the duodenal wall

Direct measurement of the thickness of the duodenal wall, either by computed tomography or magnetic resonance examination, is one of the most reliable indicators that show the damage of the duodenal wall, regardless of whether it is a neoplastic invasion or an inflammatory reaction (**Figure 8**).

If one compares the changes in the thickness of the duodenal wall from the duodenal tumors and the vaterian ampullomas, it is concluded that the ratio is exactly reversed, that is, in the case of the ampullomas, the probability that the duodenal wall has a normal thickness is 80%. Thus, the thickened wall raises the assumption of a primitive duodenal neoplasm more quickly than of a vaterian ampulloma but does not exclude it.

At the same time, the analysis of the dimensions of the parietal thickening according to the classification in the three subgroups, namely, the wall thickness with values between 4–6, 6–8, and over 8 mm, will show that in the case of the vaterian ampullomas, the wall can be thickened only up to 6 mm.

In conclusion, in the case of an ampullary neoplasia besides the fact that the probability of the presence of a thick duodenal wall is relatively small, in less than one fifth of cases, this thickening is minimal, the duodenal wall not exceeding 6 mm, as opposed to the duodenal malignancies in which at least in two-thirds of the cases we encountered a parietal thickening of more than 6 mm.

Also, the parietal thickening, in the case of neoplasms of the ampulla of Vater, has been shown to be unilateral, so it is an impairment of the duodenal wall through contiguity and at the same time limited.

The measurement of the parietal thickness is done either within the CT scan or by magnetic resonance scan, the results being identical [1, 21, 22].

3.8 Tumor extension

As with parietal thickening, the study of tumoral extension, either by contiguity, or by lymphatic or blood route, of the vaterian ampullomas is carried out by the

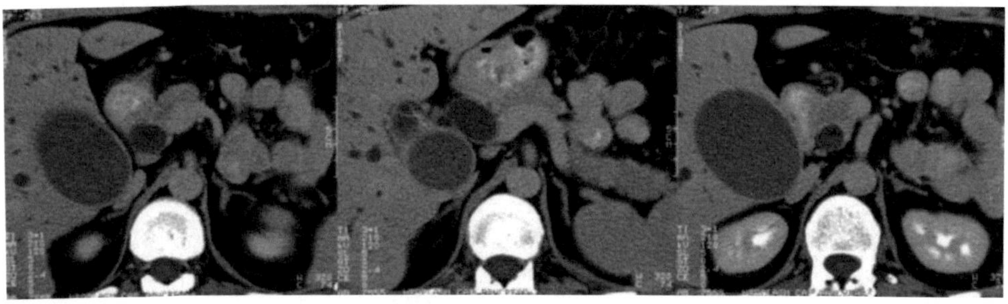

Figure 8.
Duodenal parietal change in the papilla.

two radioimaging methods, namely, computed tomography and magnetic resonance imaging. The comparative results of the two methods proved to be identical.

The extension by contiguity, in the case of the ampullary neoplasms, consisted in reality only in the invasion of the pancreatic cephalic portion, the periduodenal space, as we described in the previous subchapters being normal.

Invasion of the head of the pancreas can be detected only in up to 20% of patients with vaterian ampulloma.

If we compare the existing data with those described in the case of the primitive duodenal malignancies, it can be observed that the numbers and the percentages of pancreatic invasions in the case of duodenal neoplasms are higher than the results in the case of the vaterian ampulloma. Thus, duodenal malignancies invade the pancreas in about 30% of cases, while in the case of ampullar carcinoma, this percentage is only 20%. This is an additional argument to support the idea that the vaterian ampulloma is a less aggressive form of neoplasm, even more "benign" than primitive duodenal malignancies.

The lymphatic extension results in radio-imagistic findings of adenopathy. In specialized literature, they are described as being possibly present in the case of vaterian ampullomas, as claimed by Semelka et al. [19], but they are extremely rare.

Extension through the bloodstream is evidenced by the presence of organ metastases, respectively located in the liver. Semelka et al. [19] describes the possibility of the existence of liver metastases in the case of the vaterian ampulloma.

The frequency of metastasis in ampullary neoplasms has been shown to be lower than in the case of primitive duodenal malignancies.

In conclusion, the vaterian ampullomas are neoplasms with reduced aggression, which is why Talamini et al. [2] state that compared to pancreatic carcinomas, ampullary carcinomas have a significantly higher resectability rate and a much better prognosis.

3.9 Modifications of the biliary and pancreatic ducts

If, in the case of the duodenal neoplasms, the impairment of the bile ducts was only limited to the increase of the choledoch caliber in a few cases, the dilation in these cases was moderate, that is, it did not exceed 1.5 cm; in the situation of the vaterian ampullae, an enlargement of the bile duct tree size is detected in all cases.

In order to be able to classify the caliber changes of the biliary ducts, we divided the cases into three groups, namely, those with a diameter of less than 1.5 cm, but over 0.9 cm, those with diameters between 1.5 and 2 cm, and those with a caliber of over 2 cm.

The value of 0.9 cm is considered by all authors to be the maximum value of the choledoch duct that can be considered normal.

It can be seen that most of the vaterian ampullomas, that is to say, 70% have a choledoch with a size between 1.5 and 2 cm and over 20% with a size of over 2 cm. A percentage of less than 10% shows a moderate increase in the size of the choledoch duct, i.e., up to 1.5 cm [1] (**Figure 9a, b**).

Semelka et al. [19] concluded that most of the neoplasms of the ampulla of Vater are defined by a significant increase in the size of the choledoch duct, considered by him to be over 1.5 cm, and that only in a limited number of cases does the choledochal dilation not exceed 1.5 cm.

Regarding the radioimaging method for determining the dimensions of the choledoch duct, the same author, in a comparative study, concludes that the magnetic resonance scan, which also includes cholangio-MRI, is superior to the computed tomography, especially due to its ability to detect once again very small processes of

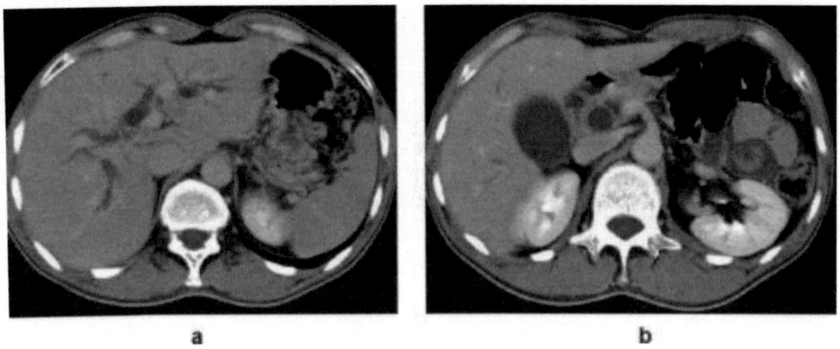

Figure 9.
(a, b) Changes of bile ducts in the vaterian ampulloma.

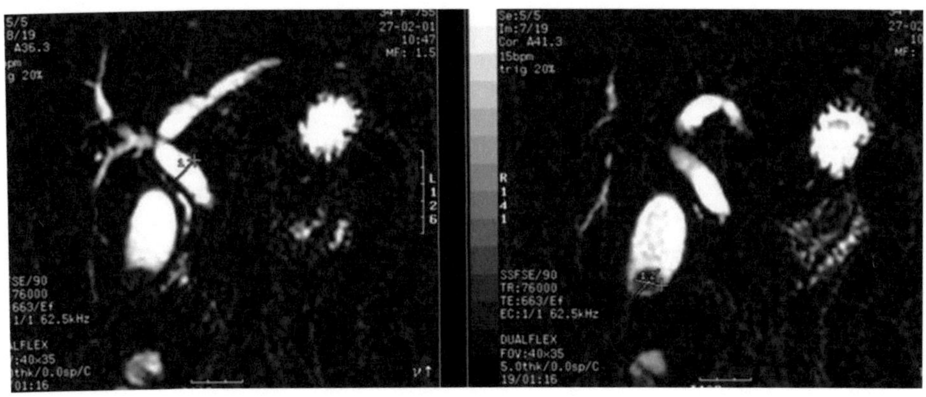

Figure 10.
Changes in the bile duct in the ampulloma: Cholangio-MRI.

space replacement at the level of the ampulla of Vater, which are not evidenced by the computed tomographic examination. He also argues that the magnetic resonance method is similar to ERCP from these points of view, but unlike the latter it is a noninvasive method.

If we compare it with the neoplasms of the head of the pancreas, we will notice that the dilation of the choledoch duct is reduced in terms of caliber, that is, in the case of pancreatic cephalic malignancies, the frequency of the presence of the choledoch dilation is much lower, of only about 30%, and dimensionally the choledoch rarely exceeds 1.5 cm.

Magnetic resonance exploration at the same time allows the study of the contours of the terminal part of the choledoch (**Figure 10**).

The existence of an irregular contour, particular to a neoplastic infiltration, cannot be discussed, considering that the Oddi sphincter usually represents an anatomical barrier in the superior extension of the tumor. The association of the terminal part of the choledoch narrowing with its irregular contours guides the diagnosis either toward a distal cholangiocarcinoma or in the case of a choledochal invasion by a pancreatic neoplasm.

This is the reason why the analysis of changes in the biliary duct was limited to dimensional evaluation.

Due to the anatomical position, the ampullar neoplasm also determines the dilation of the duct of Wirsung but only in a third of the cases. Semelka et al. [19] considers the presence of a high-caliber Wirsung as a nonspecific sign, accompanying the choledochal dilation, in a ratio similar to that found in our study.

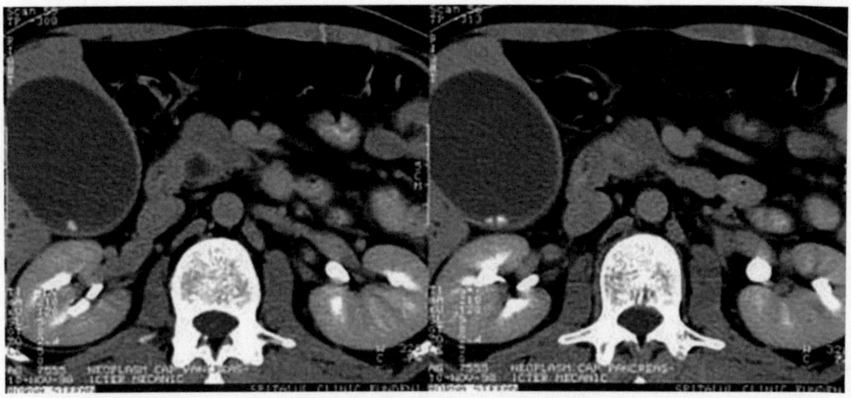

Figure 11.
Lithiasis and bladder distension associated with a vaterian ampulloma.

3.10 Changes in the gallbladder

In the case of the vaterian ampullomas, changes of the gallbladder can also occur, namely, in volume, wall, as well as the presence of calcifications inside (**Figure 11**).

The changes of the gallbladder are detected by computed tomography or magnetic resonance in 33% of occurrences in the case of the vaterian ampullomas, but without being able to distinguish if they were preexisting or caused by neoplasia [1].

Comparing to primitive duodenal neoplasms, there are no changes to the cholecyst.

It is considered that over 60% of the changes of the gallbladder in the tumor pathology of the duodenopancreatic region are detected in the cases of neoplasms of the ampulla of Vater. This leads to the conclusion that the presence of a gap in the periampullary region associated with changes in the choledochal caliber and with changes in the cholecyst leads the diagnosis to a vaterian ampulloma.

It is considered that there are no intracholecystic tumor masses and that the presence of vesicular lithiasis predominated in the case of the vaterian ampullomas.

In the case of ampullary carcinomas, there is no analysis of the changes of the vessels, due to their nonexistence, taking into account the anatomical reports of the ampulla of Vater.

4. Differential diagnosis

The vaterian ampulloma is a neoplastic entity with precise diagnostic elements, which reduces the list of possible differential diagnoses.

By anatomical topography, the only possible differential diagnoses are pancreatic neoplasm and duodenal malignancy.

For both diagnoses the role of CT and MRI is defined.

Pancreatic head neoplasm:

With the help of CT, but especially MRI, it is established from the beginning the location of the tumor mass, the size, the changes in structure, and the contrast of the pancreatic cephalic tumor mass. MRCP contributes to the analysis of changes in the biliary tree and duct of Wirsung, specific to pancreatic cephalic neoplasm.

Diagnostic elements from conventional radiological examination are not practically discussed.

Malignant duodenal tumors:

Historically, there were conventional radiological signs, most of them indirect, to suspect a malignant duodenal tumor.

Basically, the real differential diagnosis is made using CT/MRI examination.

Duodenal parietal changes, luminal stenosis, localization, structural analysis, and contrast enhancement are defining elements in establishing the diagnosis of duodenal malignancy.

Abbreviations

CT	computed tomography
MRCP	magnetic resonance cholangiopancreatography
MRI	magnetic resonance imaging
IV	intravenous
ERCP	endoscopic retrograde cholangiopancreatography
D2	descending duodenum

Author details

Ana Magdalena Bratu[1,2] and Constantin Zaharia[1,2*]

1 Department of Radiology and Medical Imaging, "Colțea" Clinical Hospital, Bucharest, Romania

2 "Carol Davila" University of Medicine and Pharmacy, Bucharest, Romania

*Address all correspondence to: czaharia50@gmail.com

References

[1] Bratu AM, Cristian D. Tumori duodenale Consideratii Imagistice si Endoscopice. Bucuresti: Universitara Carol Davila; 2014

[2] Talamini MA, Moesinger RC, Pitt HA, Sohn TA, Hruban RH, Lillemoe KD, et al. Adenocarcinoma of the ampulla of Vater. A 28-year experience. Annals of Surgery. 1997;**225**(5):590-599; Discussion 599-600

[3] Balthazar EJ. CT of the small bowel obstruction. AJR. 1994;**162**:255-261

[4] Baron RL, Stanley RJ, Lee JKT, et al. Computed tomographic features of biliary obstruction. AJR. 1983;**140**:1173-1178

[5] van Beers B, Pringot J, Trigaux JP, Jonard P, Collard JM. La tomodensitometrie de l'oesophage, de l'estomac et du duodenum. Journal of the Belgian Society of Radiology. 1989;**72**:75

[6] Buthiau D. TDM et IRM Cliniques. Paris: Frison-Roche; 1991

[7] Dudiak KM, Johnson CD, Stephens DH. Primary tumors of the small intestine: CT evaluation. AJR. 1989;**152**:995

[8] Sugi MD, Menias CO, Lubner MG, Bhalla S, Mellnick VM, Kwon MH. Katz DSCT findings of acute small-bowel entities. Radiographics. 2018;**38**(5):1352-1369. DOI: 10.1148/rg.2018170148

[9] Dudea S, Badea R. Ecografiespecială. Cluj Napoca: UMF; 1998

[10] Maccioni F, Martinelli M, Al Ansari N, Kagarmanova A, De Marco V, Zippi M, et al. Resonance cholangiography: Past, present and future: A review. European Review for Medical and Pharmacological Sciences. 2010;**14**:721-725

[11] Matos C, Metens T, Devière J, Nicaise N, Braudé P, Van Yperen G, et al. Pancreatic duct: Morphologic and functional evaluation with dynamic MR pancreatography after secretin stimulation. Radiology. 1997;**203**:435-441

[12] Lee NJ, Kim KW, Kim TK, Kim MH, Kim SY, Park MS, et al. Secretin-stimulated MRCP. Abdominal Imaging. 2006;**31**:575-581

[13] Boraschi P, Donati F, Gigoni R, Odoguardi F, Neri E, Boggi U, et al. Pancreatic transplants: Secretin-stimulated MR pancreatography. Abdominal Imaging. 2007;**32**:207-214

[14] Cappeliez O, Delhaye M, Devière J, Le Moine O, Metens T, Nicaise N, et al. Chronic pancreatitis: Evaluation of pancreatic exocrine function with MR pancreatography after secretin stimulation. Radiology. 2000;**215**:358-364

[15] Zuccaro P, Stevens T, Repas K, Diamond R, Lopez R, Wu B, et al. Magnetic resonance cholangiopancreatography reports in the evaluation of chronic pancreatitis: A need for quality improvement. Pancreatology. 2009;**9**:764-769

[16] Soto JA, Alvarez O, Lopera JE, Múnera F, Restrepo JC, Correa G. Biliary obstruction: Findings at MR cholangiography and cross-sectional MR imaging. Radiographics. 2000;**20**:353-366

[17] Katabathina VS, Dasyam AK, Dasyam N, Hosseinzadeh K. Adult bile duct strictures: Role of MR imaging and MR cholangiopancreatography in characterization. Radiographics.

2014;**34**(3):565-586. DOI: 10.1148/rg.343125211

[18] Caroli J, Soupalt R, Kossakowski J, et al. La dilatation polycystique congenitaledes voles biliaires intrahepatiques: Essai de classification. Semaine des Hôpitaux de Paris. 1958;**34**:488

[19] Semelka RC, Kelekis NL, Gesine J, Ascher SM, Burdeny D, Siegelman ES. Ampullary carcinoma: Demonstration by current MR Techniques. JMRI. 1997;7:153-156

[20] Ferruci JT. Chapter 25: The postbulbar duodenum. In: Radiology. Vol. 4. Philadelphia, USA: Lippincott-Raven; 1998

[21] Nikolaidis P, Hammond NA, Day K, Yaghmai V, Wood CG 3rd, Mosbach DS, et al. Imaging features of benign and malignant ampullary and periampullary lesions. Radiographics. 2014;**34**(3):624-641. DOI: 10.1148/rg.343125191. Review

[22] Barykov VN. Diagnosis and surgical treatment of tumors in pancreatoduodenal area. Khirurgiia (Mosk). 2000;**10**:20-23